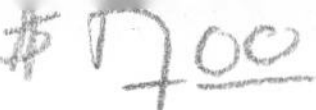

Time Bomb from Within

Mercury Poisoning in Dentistry

Dr. Stuart Scheckner

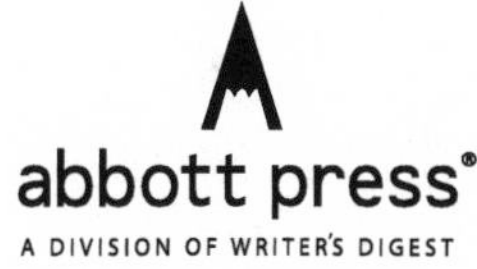

Time Bomb from Within
Mercury Poisoning in Dentistry

Abbott Press books may be ordered through booksellers or by contacting:

Abbott Press
1663 Liberty Drive
Bloomington, IN 47403
www.abbottpress.com
Phone: 1-866-697-5310

ISBN: 978-1-4582-0589-6 (sc)
ISBN: 978-1-4582-0588-9 (e)

Library of Congress Control Number: 2012915978

Printed in the United States of America

Abbott Press rev. date: 10/22/2012

Comments from Noted Authorities

"I have read your book and found it compelling and worthy of publication. It tells a sordid story about the USA's medical regulatory agencies total lack of honesty in evaluating a product that is making a major profit for those who know how to use lobbyists to make all the rules and laws in their favor."

Boyd E. Haley, PhD
Professor Emeritus of Chemistry/Biochemistry of the University of Kentucky, Chair of Chemistry for 8 years between 1997-2005,
Fellow of the IAOMT (FIAOMT)

"Dr. Scheckner's book gives the reader a close-up look at how dangerous mercury in dentistry can be to dentists, not just to the patients. Dentistry is perhaps the most dangerous profession, with the occupational exposure due to the breathing in of fine amalgam particles and mercury vapor. Contrary to the ADA's propaganda, a large fraction of dentists are, in fact, becoming mercury poisoned. This book is a wake-up call to them: doctor, your life is on the line!"

Leo Cashman, Executive Director
DAMS, Dental Amalgam Mercury Solutions

"A worthy book to read . . . A worthy lesson from a personal experience!"

Louis W. Chang, PhD
Noted researcher, scholar, and author in metal toxicology

"Dr. Stuart Scheckner has written a vital book that will help anyone on their road to improved health. He documents how amalgam fillings are impairing the health of the population. He questions why dental amalgams are still being promoted as a safe dental material when so much scientific evidence exists to the contrary. Following his life story and experience with mercury provides us all with irrefutable evidence that mercury exposure is affecting the lives of so many people. Dental Amalgams adverse health effects are still widely ignored by mainstream medicine that ignore causes and just prescribe drugs to mask symptoms."

Garry F. Gordon, MD, DO, MD(H)
Founder/President of the International College of Advanced Longevity (ICALM), internationally recognized expert on chelation therapy, Board Member of International Oxidative Medicine Association (IOMA), Co-Founder of the American College for Advancement in Medicine (ACAM)

"This is a compelling story of Dr. Scheckner's total health collapse due to his and our dental profession's total lack of understanding about the toxicity of mercury and his lifelong effort to recover. This book's beautifully detailed report of one person's odyssey will surely help countless others who continue to suffer because they have not yet discovered their mouth is the source of their health problems."

David Kennedy, DDS
Past President of the International Academy of Oral Medicine and Toxicology

"Dr. Scheckner has presented what I call a Diary of Disaster truly from his heart. Having lived some of what he experienced, I am amazed that he with-held his true feelings about how our profession puts personal liability before patient and dentist disaster. Perhaps the public can see the truth of the matter and avoid the diseases and conditions that are inherent in exposure to such vile toxins."

Hal A. Huggins DDS, MS
Immunology and Toxicology, Noted author and lecturer

Contents

About the Author

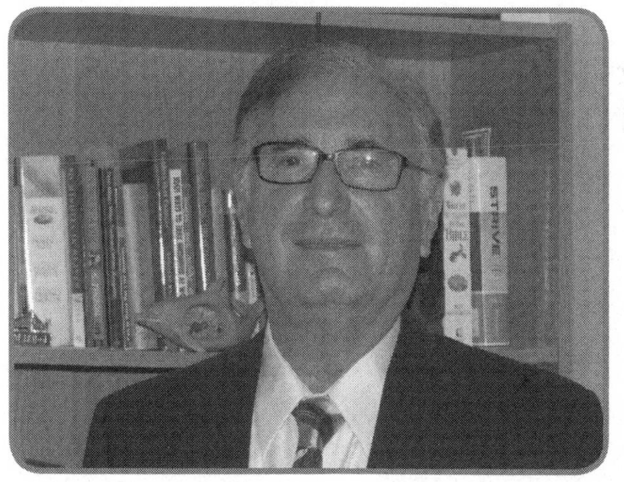

Dr. Stuart Scheckner received both his bachelor of science (1960) and doctor of dental medicine (1964) degrees from Fairleigh Dickinson University in Teaneck, New Jersey. Upon graduation, he served two years at MacDill Air Force Base in Tampa, Florida, as a captain at their dental clinic. In 1972 he moved with his family to Sarasota, Florida, where he opened a dental practice on beautiful Siesta Key.

He was living his dream: a rewarding and successful dental practice, a loving wife and two healthy children, and a waterfront home. He was a respected member of the community and had many good friends and all the amenities of a good life that money could buy.

Then it all began to change. What started subtly as some symptoms common with stress, evolved into a life-threatening ordeal, taking him on a roller-coaster ride through physical, mental, and emotional turmoil. There were times that he stood alone in his suffering, without any support, understanding, or hope of recovery. Yet, somehow, he pulled himself through it all.

Dr. Scheckner's desire to find meaning to all that has happened to him over the past thirty years has driven him to speak out on what he truly believes is a national tragedy. His interests in medicine, nutrition, and health have guided him in his search for the truth about the effect of mercury in dentistry and in our environment. He has written many letters to legislators and the press about the danger of mercury in dentistry. He is published in the Journal of Clinical Pharmacy with a pediatric immunologist on mercury associated with autoimmune disorders. He has appeared on local television and radio talk shows. His story appeared several times in featured newspaper articles. He was an expert consultant to the Florida State Board of Dentistry and was an instructor for dental assistants.

His goal in Time Bomb from Within is to question why something as insidious as mercury is still being approved for use today. He wants the public to be informed about the toxic effect of mercury in dental amalgams.

His desire is to enlighten both public officials and health professionals on the hazard of low level sub-acute chronic mercury exposure as a contributor and possible cause of many health problems. To accomplish this gives meaning to all he has endured.

Dedicated to the millions of people who have suffered mercury exposure from their mercury-silver dental fillings[1]

The journey that I take you on in this book is one that you, a family member, or a friend may face! I hope it gives you insight into this hidden problem, how to deal with it, and protect your family.

G. Mark Richardson, PhD, "one of the world's best known risk assessment specialists has provided a new risk assessment for dental amalgam fillings. His finding was that an estimated 122 million Americans are at an unacceptable level of risk from the mercury vapor levels from their dental amalgam mercury fillings!"[2]

1 Mark Richardson, *Dental Truth,* (April 2011): 15.

2 *Ibid.*

In Memoriam
Dr. Michael Ziff

After Dr. Hal Huggins announced at his seminar in Orlando that mercury was leaking out of the common silver dental filling, Dr. Ziff exclaimed to me, "Oh my God, I've been poisoning my patients!"

I hope that through my story, I can raise public awareness of the danger of mercury exposure in any form and follow through with what Dr. Michael Ziff has begun.

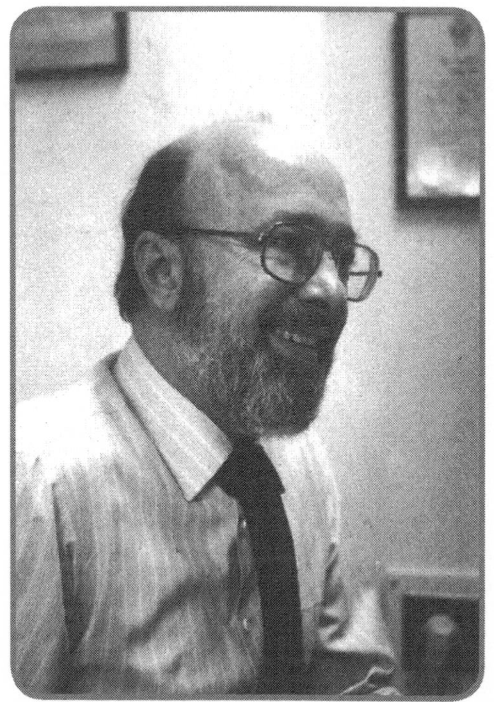

Michael Ziff, DDS

August 17, 1937 – April 22, 2004

Dr. Michael Ziff was a driving force in the formation of the International Academy of Oral Medicine and Toxicology (IAOMT).

Acknowledgements

I am grateful for the assistance of:

- Dr. David Kennedy
  Former president of the International Academy of Oral Medicine and Toxicology

And

- Leo Cashman
  Executive Director DAMS, Dental Amalgam Mercury Solutions
  Editor of Dental Truth

Disclaimer

This book is an expression of my opinion. The facts in this book are presented to the best of my knowledge. It is a biography of what happened to me as a dentist and an exposé of the hidden danger of mercury.

An asterisk is used on the first mention of an anonymous name. An anonymous name may not be used to suggest an identity.

The information in this book is not designed to give you a diagnosis or to treat an illness. The evaluations and other materials presented in this book are for informational purposes only, and are not intended to substitute for medical or mental health advice. Please consult a licensed medical practitioner qualified in this area of medicine.

Preface

Someday, future generations will look back on twentieth century dentistry. They shall say, "How could it be possible that people were having mercury, a deadly poison, implanted in their teeth?"

I am a dentist. I was poisoned from a large spill of mercury hidden in a deep shag carpet in my dental office. Mercury is recognized as an occupational hazard to dentists. However, its use in mercury-silver fillings is claimed by organized dentistry to be generally safe. The story that you are about to read is true.

<u>Mercury-Silver Fillings</u>
(Dental Amalgams)

A mercury-silver filling is a common restoration that has been used in dentistry for over 160 years. This filling is also known as a dental amalgam. Generally the public has given little thought to this material thinking it was just silver. However, about *50 percent of this filling is actually mercury, a deadly poison.* Since 1979, a raging controversy has developed regarding the safety of this material. This book is unique and different from many books on this subject. I am a mercury poisoned dentist, and through my eyes, you will see the agony and frustration I endured dealing with the medical and legal systems. From my story, you will gain a new insight into the dental amalgam controversy.

As a practicing general dentist, I became disabled because of mercury toxicity. I went through years of agony without a clue of what was happening to me. The physicians whom I had seen were just as clueless.

It wasn't until I read a document by chemistry Professor Alfred Stock, from 1926, that I was able to relate my symptoms to mercury exposure. Stock experimented extensively with mercury at that time, wrote about it in great detail, and went on to lead an international crusade against the use of mercury-silver (amalgams) fillings in dentistry. As I read his research paper and the description of his symptoms of mercury poisoning, chills went through my body as I suddenly realized that my own suffering was due to mercury.

This was the start of my quest to learn about mercury toxicity and understand what had happened to me. I researched books at the local medical hospital library. I read and compiled hundreds of pages of documents about mercury. I published an article in the *Journal of Clinical Pharmacy* with a pediatric immunologist, Michael McCann, MD.

The diagnosis of my mercury toxicity was validated by one of the leading world mercury toxicologists, Professor Louis Chang. He paid me a compliment once: he facetiously said that I deserved a PhD in mercury toxicology. Then, I asked him why *physicians* have such a poor knowledge of mercury toxicity. He said that the medical curriculum is so intense that little time is available for that.

The effect of mercury exposure is not all-or-nothing. There are varying degrees of health effects due to such variables as genetic susceptibility to being poisoned, amount of mercury one is exposed to, presence of infections, and other toxic exposures. Because of the extremely insidious nature of mercury toxicity, you can easily have a mercury induced-problem and attribute it to something else. In addition, it is extremely difficult to diagnose chronic sub-acute mercury toxicity as a factor. In other words, you cannot rule out mercury if there is any reason to believe a person has been exposed to mercury in some way, such as from mercury-silver fillings.

With my devastating experience with mercury toxicity as a dentist, I feel compelled to inform my fellow dentists, as well as physicians, and dental patients of this dangerous poison. I have talked to many of my dental colleagues and have found that they have very limited knowledge of mercury toxicity. We dentists are exposed to one of the most toxic and dangerous materials known to man. If you place or remove dental amalgams and you lack the very elaborate protections that are needed, then you, the dentist, are being exposed to dangerous levels of mercury vapor!

In my search for the truth of what happened to me, I came across something so shocking. Mercury, the same poison that poisoned me, is a nemesis of mankind. Dentistry has implanted this insidious deadly poison in hundreds of millions of people. Mercury was not locked into the filling material as we had been told for over a century. It contaminates the human body. The poisonous mercury vapors escape and accumulate in vital organs, such as the kidney, the GI tract, the liver, and the brain. Go with me on my search for the truth and my quest to recover my health.

Since the article by Professor Stock made such an impression on me, I am including excerpts from it:

"The Dangerousness of Mercury Vapor"
Professor Alfred Stock, PhD, 1926

> "There is no doubt that many complaints such as fatigue, memory weakness, oral inflammation, diarrhea, lack of appetite, chronic runny nose and sinusitis are sometimes caused by mercury that has been directed to the body from amalgam fillings, maybe only in small quantities, but constantly. The physicians should give this fact the most serious attention. Then it will probably become apparent that the frivolous introduction of amalgams as a tooth filling device was a nasty sin against humanity.
>
> Insidious mercury poisonings are certainly much more common than ordinarily thought."

Introduction

General dentists work with mercury. This liquid metal is one of the most toxic substances known to man. Mercury is much more toxic than lead, cadmium, and arsenic. Some authorities, in fact, say that no amount of exposure to mercury vapor can be considered totally harmless. The question is, should we be concerned? Is the danger real?

Most dentists are not aware of the symptoms of mercury toxicity. The objective of this book, hence, is to inform my fellow dentists, my medical colleagues, and the public of the real dangers of exposure to mercury. Mercury is an extremely dangerous and insidious poison!

Dentists are occupationally exposed to mercury vapor. Exposure especially happens while placing or removing amalgams, unless elaborate protections are used. Mercury is primarily neuro-toxic and secondarily immuno-toxic. It not only affects the nervous system, but also harms the immune, endocrine, reproductive, and digestive systems. Therefore, it is in our best interest to avoid any mercury exposure or at least reduce it.

Studies have been performed on dental personnel demonstrating neuro-behavioral deficits. Dentists who are occupationally exposed to mercury exhibit a below-normal score on motor speed, visual scanning, verbal and visual memories, and visuomotor coordination.[3]

---

[3] *Source: Ngim, CH; et al., "Chronic Neurobehavioral Effects of Elemental Mercury in Dentists," Brit J Indust Med, 1992, 49:782-90.*

In another report, the mercury level in the urinary mercury excretion of dentists was higher as a group, confirming increased exposure. "Analysis of data revealed that neuro-psychological, muscular, respiratory, cardiovascular, and dermal symptoms were more prevalent in dentists. Our findings indicate that occupational exposure of dentists to mercury, even at low levels, is associated with a significant increase in the prevalence of symptoms of intoxication." [4]

> "PMS and infertility are common among many young female dental workers due at least in part to their mercury exposure. Male dental workers also suffer from infertility. Mercury lowers zinc levels, which in turn leads to lower testosterone (male hormone) levels."[5]

Metallic mercury vaporizes. Approximately 80 percent of the vapor is absorbed through the lungs. Within minutes, the uncharged ion crosses the blood-brain barrier. In the brain, the mercury changes into a charged ion. Now, the blood brain-barrier does not allow its release, so an accumulation occurs in the brain.

Liquid mercury is the inorganic form of mercury that is mixed with a silver mixture to form an amalgam. Inorganic mercury can be transformed in the body by methylation into an even more toxic organic form of mercury, methylmercury. This occurs because of intestinal bacteria and yeasts.[6], [7] In another study, it was found that mouth bacteria could methylate mercury into the more dangerous methylmercury.[8]

---

4 Masoud NEGHAB, Alireza CHOOBINEH, Jafar HASSAN ZADEH, Ebrahim GHADERI, "Symptoms of Intoxication in Dentists Associated with Exposure to Low Levels of Mercury", Industrial Health 2011, 49, 249-254.

5 *William R. Kellas, PhD and Andrea Sharon Dworkin, N.D,. "Surviving the Toxic Crisis", 1996, p.188.*

6 T. Edwards and B. C. McBride, *Nature* 253 (1975): 24.

7 I. R. Rowland, P. Grasso, and M. J. Davies, "The Methylation of Mercury Chloride by Human Intestinal Bacteria," *Experientia* 31 (1975): 1064–1065.

8 U. Heintze et al., "Methylation of Mercury from Dental Amalgam and Mercuric Chloride by Oral Streptococci In Vitro," *Scand J Dent Res* 91, no. 2 (1983): 150–152.

With regard to the occupational safety of the use of mercury in our dental practice, the A.D.A. (American Dental Association) has given us guidelines to follow such as the storage of waste dental amalgam. At some of the dental conventions, urine mercury tests were made available. In this book, you will find that urine mercury levels are not necessarily diagnostic of mercury toxicity. It is possible to have the symptoms of mercury toxicity with urine mercury levels that are low or virtually zero.

Since mercury has been a part of general practice, dentists need to know the risks involved in its use. Removing an amalgam has even greater risk of mercury exposure to the dentist than placing an amalgam. When grinding out an old amalgam, a large amount of mercury particles is released into the air, which the dentist and the patient can breathe in.

The information in this book was learned the hard way. I lost a major part of my dental career and almost died from exposure to mercury. If I had not taken a course or read some information on the subject, I would not have found out what had happened to me. I believe that most dental patients do not know that they are being exposed to mercury from their silver fillings and that it could have an impact on their health.

I have spoken to a number of dentists with disabling mercury toxicity. Such a sad development is commonplace in dentistry, contrary to ADA claims, and these dentists' symptoms, caused by their mercury exposure, show remarkable similarities.

The bits and pieces of information that will be presented herein are published facts and research on mercury exposure and show that there is no level of exposure that is safe. In fact, the diagnosis of chronic mercury toxicity in general is poorly understood. It has been my experience, as well as others, that an average physician cannot diagnose chronic mercury toxicity if it were right in front of him. I am a living proof of that. I must have seen at least a dozen physicians. After reading this book, a physician will understand that it is almost impossible to rule out mercury as a cause of mental, neurological, neuro-psychological, and immunological health problems. If there is any type of known mercury exposure, it should be considered as a possible factor.

By reading "Time Bomb from Within", you will learn the truth about the insidious nature of mercury exposure. The motto "What you don't know can hurt you," applies here.

Chapter 1

Early Years

Back in the 1940's, mass commercialism had not set in yet. My family lived in the Bronx. The trolley traversed the road in front of our apartment building on Bronx Park East. We did not need a car to get around. I walked to the elementary school. We could walk to our grocery store in just a few minutes.

As a young boy in the1940's, I remember the old time grocery store. There were no giant supermarkets at the time. The butter was stored in the form of a large cube in the refrigerator. The grocer would cut off a piece for us and place it in wax paper. What I especially remember about this butter is that when you bought it in the winter, it had a very light color, just about white. When you bought the butter in the summer, it was a very deep yellow. This had to do with the fact that the cows ate hay in the winter and grass in the summer. It was natural.

Today, foods abound with all kinds of chemicals. It is hard to find food products that are not processed. Foods are canned, hydrogenated, dehydrated and reconstituted, irradiated, and preserved with many different chemicals. This is necessary to be able to supply the demand for foods. Yet, there is a price for this that is indeed very subtle. We are subjecting the population to a massive experiment. Each chemical additive in itself may not be proven harmful in the amount normally consumed, but what happens when you add the plethora of chemicals together? Do we really know?

Surely, it would be hard to conclude that the storage of chemicals in the body is completely safe. Even DDT, which is now banned, can still be found in the fat tissues of senior citizens today. Many chemicals have a long half-life. That means it takes so many years for the chemical to be reduced in half in the body. Mercury in the brain has a half-life of up to thirty-two years (this amount differs greatly because of individual variation). This is a sobering thought for anyone exposed to mercury. You may think, well, who is exposed to mercury, which is one of the deadliest toxic materials known to man? Do you know anyone who has mercury poisoning? I did not until…

Chapter 2

Finally Graduated

I graduated from Fair Lawn High School in New Jersey in 1956 and started college the next year. Commuting to New York University was a hassle, so the following year, I decided to take the dental program of Fairleigh Dickinson University in Teaneck, New Jersey which was much closer to my home. At Fairleigh Dickinson University, I attended both the undergraduate and postgraduate dental programs.

My dad had wanted me to take up medicine, and I would have been a good MD, but practicality ruled my life. My decision to be a dentist was based on such practicality as working on good hours and not being constantly on call.

So the decision had been made to enter the dental profession. Dr. Peter Sammartino, the president of the university, welcomed our freshman dentistry class. He said that of any profession, dentistry emphasizes preventive care. In other words, we try to help patients have a healthy mouth, thereby lessening the need for our services. We are indeed in a very noble profession.

Eight long years of college were finally over. It was 1964. Finally graduating dental school was a huge accomplishment. It had taken me years of study and hard work to earn my degree in dentistry. On the lighter side, after graduation, my grandmother, in her Yiddish accent, said, "So vie didn't you become a real doctor?"

Our graduating dentistry class of 1964 was given the opportunity to sign up for military services. I opted for the Air Force.

There were forty-eight students in our graduating class, and most of us opted to go into military service. The majority was accepted to the army dental program, only one to the Navy, and two to the Air Force. I was excited that I made it to the Air Force. It was a momentous day that I left Fair Lawn, New Jersey in my 1959 Chevrolet Impala and started my trip to Alabama for my Air Force orientation program. After several weeks of orientation into the Air Force, I was sent to MacDill Air Force Base in Tampa, Florida. It was great!

It was the first time I was down South. The weather was beautiful. I was a captain in the Air Force. My practice of dentistry was fulfilling. It was like an internship. I had to treat many different problems, and it was a great "esprit de corps" having the comradeship of fellow dentists.

My two-year tour in the Air Force was perhaps the best years of my life. I got married during this time. My wife and I were perpetual tourists in Florida. Every weekend, we would be off discovering a different highlight of Florida's vacation wonderland from Busch Gardens, to Weeki Wachee Springs, Cypress Gardens, Sunken Gardens, and the list goes on.

The clinic had about twelve dentists. One year, under the direction of Colonel Bennett, we were the most productive clinic in the Air Force. I was able to intern in the prosthetic and the oral surgery programs. Colonel Bennett was a smart man in giving us that option. I felt that I wanted to stay in Florida. But then, I would need a Florida dental license. There were three other dentists who wanted to take the state board. In a nutshell, I felt lucky to be the only one dentist out of the four dentists from our base to pass the exam. Relatively, not many dentists received dental licenses that year. The exam was given in a hotel ballroom without any dental facilities.

There was no air conditioning and the heat made the wax soft and difficult to work with in making a denture setup. It was easy to lose your cast gold inlay in a large barrel of water filled with debris when you quenched the hot casting ring. You had to use your own slow speed cord driven handpiece (dental drill) for tooth preparations on a live patient. There was no aspiration (suction) for saliva. Florida dentists today are fortunate to have their dental exams in a modern facility. Indeed, I was lucky to have passed the exam in this huge hotel ballroom without dental facilities.

Well, the big decision of whether to stay in Florida was drawing near. It was 1966. My two-year tour in the Air Force was almost over. Dr. Martinez, a local dentist, offered me one of his vacant buildings plumbed for a dental office. Perhaps I felt guilty about living away from my parents or starting on my own so far away from New Jersey. My wife wanted to stay in Florida. However, I opted to go back to New Jersey. Perhaps the story detailed in this book would not have happened if I opened my own practice in Florida at that time instead of going back to New Jersey.

For the next six years in New Jersey, we dreamed of going back to Florida. One night, my car got stuck in the ice and snow near my office in Garfield, New Jersey. This was the last straw; I decided we were going back to Florida. Until that time, I had just made calls to inquire about dental practices in Florida. Now, we were going to drive down to Florida. We arrived in Tampa and inquired about practices at a large dental supply house. None were available. Our next stop was Sarasota, about sixty miles south of Tampa along the Gulf Coast in Central Florida. This was a place we had visited several times while we were living in Tampa. We had already been to the Sarasota Jungle Gardens and the Ringling Museum of Art. We remembered Sarasota to be a very pretty area.

We arrived at a local dental supply company and spoke to the manager, Alex Suarez, about dental practices. A practice on Siesta Key on the western edge of Sarasota had just become available. I was the first dentist to find this opportunity. We saw the practice and made arrangements to buy it within six months. Six months later, we were in Florida. I took over the practice on April 1st 1972. We had found our "paradise island," Siesta Key. I was the only dentist on the key. We found a beautiful condo and had a great practice. I felt great! Everything was right with the world!

Chapter 3

Paradise Island

It seemed that things were really falling into place in my life. My timing in coming down to Florida was perfect, just when the Siesta Key dental practice had been put on the market. Siesta Key is a beautiful area. The sand on Siesta Beach is pure white, made of fine quartz. Our beach was rated as one of the nicest beaches in the world. And I was the only dentist on this paradise island. I was thirty-two years old.

Fred* and Maurine* had become very close friends. Fred was a condominium developer. We bought a condo from him overlooking Siesta Beach. It had a truly beautiful view.

This was our vacation paradise. We had people from all over the country coming to Siesta Key for vacations. My practice continued to grow and flourish. I bought a beautiful home right on a canal. I bought a twenty-two-foot boat for my weekend outings and adventures. This was indeed an exciting time of my life.

While I was practicing dentistry in New Jersey, I stood quite a lot. It took a toll on my knees. By the time I had left New Jersey for Florida, I was limping because of knee pain. The new office in Florida was set up for sit-down dentistry; so much of the time, I did not have to stand. However, the hard floor aggravated my knee problem.

I had been talking to Fred about this hard floor. I wanted to get something softer to stand on since this hard floor was causing me knee pain. Fred told me about the leftover carpeting he had from his clubroom. The carpeting he gave me was shag carpeting. It was a deep type of carpeting with long strands. Not familiar with the different types of carpeting and the appropriate carpeting for a dental office, I accepted Fred's carpeting.

It was a day in 1978. I had a busy practice. My dental assistant was out, and I needed assistance. I called my secretary, Linda*, and asked her to mix an amalgam for me. Linda was not a trained assistant. However, the procedure for mixing an amalgam is relatively simple.

This event changed my life, and the following is a description of what happened:

Although there was enough mercury in the Caulk (brand name) mercury dispensing bottle to do several fillings, Linda went to the stock room and obtained a large stock bottle of mercury. She filled the Caulk dispensing bottle with mercury to just about overflowing. I remember how the mercury was bulging just over the rim of the bottle. She then reached for the cap of the dispensing bottle, drew her arm back, and knocked the dispensing bottle onto the shag carpet beneath the dental chair. The entire content of the bottle emptied into the shag carpeting. She then proceeded to refill the Caulk dispensing bottle with mercury as if nothing had happened. Evidently, she had no idea of the danger she had placed me in. I was running behind schedule without my regular dental assistant. I remember the thought running through my mind: *I may become poisoned, but I never heard of anyone being poisoned in dentistry from mercury.* I went on to see my next patient and gave little thought to the spill after the incident except to warn all new dental assistants about the spill and remind them to be careful when handling mercury.

After I hired Susan* as my new dental assistant, we experienced a storm that drenched the carpeting in the room. The carpeting was removed at this point. By the time it was removed, the three-fourths pound of mercury had been in my carpet for at least two years. I had been exposed to the mercury in the carpet from 1978 to 1980.

Chapter 4

Seeking Help

I do not recall how much time had passed since the mercury spill before I started having very bizarre symptoms. The reason for this was that I did not identify the mercury as a problem since I had no idea what the symptoms of poisoning were. It might have been several months after the spill that I started not feeling well. As the symptoms were very insidious and very slow in coming on, it was really difficult to ascertain what the cause of my suffering was. I was experiencing some terrifying and bizarre symptoms. I could not explain what was happening to me. Perhaps I was suffering from midlife crisis or something like that. I did not know where to turn.

I have always had the highest regard for medicine. I know physicians have their limitations, but they have to be pretty good; don't they have to be? They are dealing with life-and-death situations. I think my estimation of medicine would have been better if I had not gone through my devastating experience.

I was interested in going into either medicine or dentistry. My father used to tell me that he would have liked me to go into medicine. Maybe he was right, and then this would not have happened. I chose dentistry because I did not want to be faced with life-and-death situations with a patient. I am extremely conscientious and a perfectionist and could not bear the thought of losing a patient even if it were not my fault. Dentistry offered me a profession that allowed me to help people with their health. I had my own hours unlike most medical practitioners, and I was not dealing with life and death. My work in dentistry was an art. I used to get many compliments from the specialists whom I would refer to. My patients trusted me, and they knew they were being treated kindly and gently. They knew they were getting good work. Years after I gave up my practice, I would meet many people who still remembered me and my gentle good work. Naturally, I expected this same professional expertise and care from my medical counterparts. But as it turned out, it was difficult to find a physician who could really help me. Years after my ordeal had started, I met a kind physician, Dr. Richard Sarkis, at Sarasota Memorial Hospital. My mother was just recovering from a heart problem. I talked to Dr. Sarkis in an elevator as I was about to leave the hospital. He seemed to know a little about mercury toxicity. But what he said to me that I have never forgotten is, "Psychiatry is the wastebasket of medicine." When a physician does not know what the problem is, he or she declares that it's all in the person's head; it's a mental problem.

Dr. Ray*, an internist and a cardiologist, was a friend of mine. My symptoms were not too severe when I first saw him for help. My stomach was growling constantly. The sound could be heard even without using a stethoscope. I had constant loose bowels. I had a buzz-like fine tremor in my chest and anxiety. I was looking for answers. Dr. Ray thought that I had mitral valve prolapse (benign heart disorder where the valve flaps do not work properly). He said my symptoms were experienced by some people with this problem. He sent me for an echocardiogram. The results came back negative.

Dr. Ray suggested that I work out with him at the YMCA. He thought that my problem was stress and that exercise would work it off. A person sees another person's problem through his or her own eyes. Dr. Ray was an avid bodybuilder. He went to the Y, and that's how he worked off his stress.

I mentioned the mercury spill casually to Dr. Ray. He made little of it. He said, "Forget about it, just stay away from it." Well, I did forget about it but did not stay away from it. I had kept the carpet with mercury in my treatment room a couple of years until about 1980. I had two years of exposure to a three-hundred-gram (almost three-fourths pound) mercury spill just below my dental stool. Those two years were too much and destroyed my ability to be near any work with mercury at all. Dentists work with mercury. Even if a dentist does not use dental amalgam anymore, he removes these mercury-silver fillings routinely as they break down in patients' mouths. Even with high-speed suction, thousands of 1- to 2-micron bullets shoot out of the patient's mouth with the use of a high-speed handpiece (dental drill). The revolutions per minute of a bur in a dental handpiece could be around one hundred thousand.

I asked Dr. Ray to send a letter to my friend Dr. Andrea*. Dr. Ray stated in the letter that I had seen him for an examination on April 6, 1979. Basically, it said that I had complained of stomach cramps, and that I had felt that I was suffering from exposure to free mercury in my carpeting. It also mentioned that I was suffering from indigestion and light-headed spells lasting from fifteen to twenty minutes. He also added that I was very tense and fearful and had trouble moving my feet when walking. He also explained that I was shaky at times.

Determining the urine mercury levels is very important for anyone who *recently* had a *heavy* mercury exposure. At the time of my heavy *exposure*, I had very little knowledge of mercury toxicity. Most dentists are not aware of the complexity of symptoms that accompany mercury poisoning. Unfortunately, I found out that most physicians have a very poor grasp of the subject also. Dr. Louis Chang, PhD, a foremost mercury toxicologist and a Professor at the University of Arkansas at that time, stated to me that medical students have a very intense academic curriculum, and that there is very little time for the subject of toxicity (poisoning), let alone on the part of mercury.

It is highly probable that if a urine mercury level was obtained when I had first seen Dr. Ray, it would have been high. However, the letter from Dr. Ray stated, "There was some discussion at the time about obtaining a mercury analysis, but I do not believe that was available." Of course, urine mercury testing was available and could have been performed!

Urine mercury levels are useful in showing the general exposure of a group. On an individual basis, it may show exposure but not necessarily prove toxicity.

Urine mercury testing can be useful on recent heavy exposure to mercury. A high urine mercury level indicates *exposure*, while an extremely low level of urine mercury may indicate an inability to excrete stored mercury. As time goes by, the body may lose its ability to eliminate mercury. A low urine mercury level does not rule out mercury poisoning. In fact, there are cases where urine mercury levels are high with no symptoms, and there are cases where levels of urine mercury are extremely low with symptoms. Those with symptoms and low urine mercury levels are people who are not able to detoxify and eliminate mercury from their body. As exposure continues, the stored mercury becomes greater. Therefore, a low urine mercury level does not rule out mercury poisoning when there is a possible related health problem and suspected exposure to mercury.

I was left in the lurch at this point. Years later, when mercury poisoning was suspected, there was no urine mercury level to refer to. It is like a hit-and-run driver. If you do not get the license plate of the driver, you are not going to find him or her years later. That's what I was faced with without documentation that I had high urine mercury level at that time.

Chapter 5

Grave's Disease

My dental office was located at Siesta Village Plaza on Siesta Key. Adjacent to my office was a medical office. One of the physicians from that office came over for dental work. He was a fellow dentist who went back to school and acquired his medical degree. I was talking to him about my unexplainable frightening symptoms, including my tachycardia (rapid heart rate).

He indicated that I probably had hyperthyroidism (Graves' disease) and should see an endocrinologist. I made an appointment with Dr. Herbert*, an endocrinologist. He sent me for a thyroid uptake and scan. In this procedure, a capsule of radioactive iodine is swallowed prior to the scan to measure the uptake of iodine by the thyroid. These were the results: "The thyroid uptake is abnormally increased measuring 58.6% at 24 hours." My T4 levels were very high (T4 is a hormone produced by the thyroid gland). The endocrinologist made a diagnosis of Graves' disease. This was in the year of 1982.

I was now optimistic that with a definitive diagnosis, the frightening symptoms would go away. Dr. Herbert asked me if there was a history of thyroid disease in my family as there was usually a familial tendency for it. I said no. There had never been a history of this in my family.

What was also unusual was that I did not have the typical exophthalmos (bulging eyeballs).

Dr. Herbert placed me on an anti-thyroid medication. He used Tapazole and later propylthiouracil (PTU). My T4 levels were pushed down to subnormal. Yet my symptoms did not abate and were only getting worse. With my condition worsening, Dr. Herbert assumed that I had an *anxiety problem*. He placed me on Ativan, which is used to treat anxiety disorders. Although the Ativan helped somewhat with the anxiety, my other symptoms were becoming worse.

I still could not connect my condition to the mercury exposure, which was the reason for my many symptoms and anguish. Later on, my thyroid problem's connection to mercury toxicity was made clear in a document from the World Health Organization: increased radioactive iodine uptake is one of the identifiers of mercury toxicity.

I. M. Trakhtenberg, a Russian scientist, did a study of mercury-exposed workers and found that there was a higher incidence of Graves' disease among them.

> "Studies by I.M. Trakhtenberg (1969) (reviewed by Friberg & Nordberg, 1973) indicate that exposure of rats to concentrations of elemental mercury vapour in the range of 0.1–0.3 mg/m3 for over 100 days increased uptake of radioactive iodine by the thyroid."[9]

Thus started the medical documentation, the pieces of the puzzle that needed to be put together. The diagnosis goes as far as the symptoms or the conditions caused by mercury. However, it does not go as far as finding the fundamental cause—mercury itself. Mercury can cause or be a factor in over three hundred symptoms and diseases, and yet it is most often overlooked and is not tested for properly!

---

[9] INTERNATIONAL PROGRAMME ON CHEMICAL SAFETY, ENVIRONMENTAL HEALTH CRITERIA 1, Published under the joint sponsorship of the United Nations Environment Programme and the World Health Organization World Health Organization Geneva, 1976, 7.1.2.1 Reversible damage

I was faced with medical ignorance about my condition. Each physician saw my symptoms with only the knowledge of one part of my illness. Many of the doctors whom I had seen for help saw only through their limitations and beliefs. Each sign and symptom of mercury toxicity would be taken by itself, not as part of the whole to make a diagnosis of mercury toxicity. They were seeing what was on the surface, not what was causing my condition.

Till this day, I am sure Dr. James* still sees me as a psychiatric case. Dr. James was my primary care physician from 1982 to 1984. Dr. James once placed his hand on my shoulder and said, "Stu, it will be all right, it will be all right" in a very condescending way implying that I was a psychiatric case. How humiliating! I am sure that he meant well, and he was really trying to be consoling. But this is an example of an average physician with a patient having mercury toxicity and not having a clue about it. How many people wind up in a psychiatric care unit with this kind of medical expertise when they should be treated for a toxicity problem! How profound was Dr. Richard Sarkis statement: "Psychiatry is the wastebasket of medicine." When a physician does not know what the problem is, he or she declares that it's all in the person's head; it's a mental problem.

I was not about to have a comprehensive definitive diagnosis of mercury toxicity until I flew across the United States from Florida to the state of Washington to see Sandra Denton, MD, many years later.

Chapter 6

Last Months of Practice

Siesta Key was paradise island to me. My practice was thriving as I was the only dentist on the key.

As time passed, I started feeling tired, achy, and run-down. I thought I was experiencing burnout or midlife crisis. I was tired, deathly tired. My busy practice was no longer routine. Everyday hassles were now major ordeals. I cut my hours to part-time for nearly a year. Little did I realize this was the beginning of an unbelievable nightmare.

My life had come together to live in such a paradise but was now falling apart. My dental practice was an ordeal with fatigue, internal tremors, and agitation.

I did not know where to look for answers. I called the American Dental Association, asking for help with my bizarre symptoms. They told me that there was a high suicide rate among dentists. That was comforting!

Although I remembered the spill of mercury, I did not make a connection to it. After telling Dr. Ray, my friend and internist, on a medical appointment about the mercury spill, he told me to "forget about it, just stay away from it." So I did forget about it and did not connect my symptoms to the mercury spill.

I was looking for answers. I received a flyer on a course that was being given by Dr. Hal Huggins. The course was on "body chemistry." Perhaps there was an answer for me here. After all, the doctors whom I had seen were not helping me. It was about 1981.

Dr. Huggins's course in Orlando was very informative and interesting. It was the beginning of my education on alternative medicine. Attending the course were twelve great dentists. They were on the highest level of professionalism. The course covered balancing blood chemistries, hair analysis, diet, nutrition, and overall health.

It was the third morning of Dr. Hal Huggins's seminar on body chemistry in Orlando, Florida. He had just made the dramatic announcement that mercury was leaking out of dental amalgams. He felt that amalgams would be banned as a filling material by the end of the year. This was wishful thinking as we later found out.

After the morning session, my wife and I were having lunch with Dr. Michael Ziff. It was just the three of us. Our conversation centered on the amalgam filling material that we dentists work with. This was the very "bread and butter" of dentistry. We were using a filling material that was leaking mercury! With tears in his eyes, Michael exclaimed, "Oh my God, I have been poisoning my patients!" You could feel his emotion, his care, his concern.

This was the seed of the beginning of the International Academy of Oral Medicine and Toxicology. Dr. Michael Ziff became one of the founders of this international organization that inform dentists, health professionals, and the public on the dangers posed by mercury in silver fillings.

The following is my last communication through e-mail with Dr. Michael Ziff many years later:

"Date: Fri, 1 Feb 2002 10:24:20 EST

Dear Stu:

Nice to hear from you. I am so sorry to hear of the loss of your parents. I try not to think of what I will have to go through.

We have come a long way since that fateful seminar some 20 years ago. It has been a long struggle, with many sacrifices on the part of many people. However, I do believe that we are now near victory, finally.

I certainly wish the best for you and your family.

Michael"

Perhaps it was more than coincidence that I had taken Dr. Huggins's course to find out why I was feeling so sick. I still did not have a clue. Dr. Huggins had mentioned dental amalgam but not the risk it poses to dentists, so I did not make the connection at that time. It was later that I found out that this very insidious toxic mercury was my nemesis. I had lost my dental practice in the middle of my dental career because of the very same dangerous poison that we dentists had been using in the common silver dental filling.

My symptoms continued to get worse. Then I received a newsletter containing Professor Alfred Stock's description of his ordeal with mercury toxicity. Chills went through my body as I connected my nightmare to the mercury spill.

I did a urine mercury test in 1983, five years after the mercury spill. The test came back with undetectable levels of mercury. I called Dr. Huggins about this. He explained to me that this condition was known as "retention toxicity." I called the American Dental Association. They wrote me back a letter, stating, "Don't believe the unscientific statements of 'retention toxicity', look elsewhere for your problem." This statement clearly is not consistent with research on mercury toxicity, yet this is the criterion that the ADA relies on, which excludes many people who could have low-level subacute chronic mercury toxicity. This includes dentists occupationally exposed and dental patients exposed from their mercury-silver fillings.

Now that I considered the possibility of mercury toxicity as my nemesis, I started accumulating documents on the subject, literally hundreds and hundreds of pages, including documents from medical libraries.

I hired an associate in 1983 so that I could cut down on my clinic hours. After hiring my associate, I took a month off. I started to regain my weight. No longer was I fatigued after the four weeks that I was not in the office. I felt and looked great!

Three days since I got back to the office, I was worse than ever. Within six months of only working part-time, I was in a very serious condition. I was having tachycardia, weight loss, insomnia, nausea, tremors, and metallic taste in my mouth.

Dr. Louis Chang is one of the leading mercury toxicologists in the world. He was a professor of pathology at the University of Arkansas for Medical Sciences. Dr. Chang related this story to me years later. He said he had a medical student inject rats with sublethal doses of mercuric chloride. The student was told not to skip any days. The student had to go on vacation, so the regimen of injections was put on hold. When the medical student came back from vacation and injected the rats with the sub-lethal doses of mercuric chloride, they started dying. I then related this experiment to what happened to me. After a month of no mercury exposure, my body had recovered. But then, upon my re-exposure, I was so sensitized that my reaction to low levels of mercury vapor was acute. The following is a quote from Professor Alfred Stock: "It seems that existing mercury intoxication preconditions a special sensitivity to renewed exposure from mercury vapor."

My distress and agony were becoming more acute. The last evening of my meaningful ability to perform as a dentist was most frightening. My body was shutting down. I was freezing. My body was becoming numb. I tried to keep warm under the blankets. I must have had at least five blankets on me, but I was still freezing.

The following morning, I was unable to go to my office since I was so sick. I called my physician, Dr. James. He wanted me to go to the hospital. I asked him whether they had chelation therapy for mercury. He said, "Yes". I called the hospital, and they did not have a clue about chelation for mercury. I therefore concluded that Dr. James was just trying to humor me and get me to the hospital. I later read a letter to my parents from Dr. James advising me to go to the hospital, evidently for psychiatric care. My wife adamantly told me not to go to the hospital as they would probably "kill you" with drugs. As frightened as I was with terrifying symptoms, I did not go to the hospital. This decision turned out to be the right one. Later, this decision was reinforced by gathering more information on mercury recovery and detoxification protocol and by seeing what happened to another patient, Donald*, who did go to a psychiatric ward. He had a violent reaction to the medications that he was given and had to be put in a straight jacket. Donald had many mercury-silver fillings, and he had decided to have them removed. Unfortunately, he had his fillings removed improperly causing a high exposure to mercury vapor. In addition, he had no detoxification protocol to help remove mercury from his body.

Ironically, April 1st, 1984, was the end of my dental career, 12 years to the day that I had started my practice in the Siesta Key office.

Chapter 7

My Agony of Mercury Poisoning

It is not possible to understand the unreal experience of an individual poisoned with mercury. The terror and suffering cannot be fathomed. I have gone through it! Have you ever watched a movie with psychedelic visual and sound effects? Chemicals can affect brain function. For example, LSD is a hallucinogenic drug. It can distort reality. Mercury has a profound effect on the brain. Drugs and poisons can affect the way you feel both mentally and physically.

Perhaps I was suffering from midlife crisis. All I knew was that I felt awful. My condition was hard to put into words. Even if I could put it into words somehow, it would not convey my reality of extreme suffering.

Life is truly beautiful. Nature, with its abounding beauty, surrounds us: A beautiful rose with its nectar fragrance, the air sweet from orange blossoms, a cool fresh mellow breeze. There is the love of your family—your wife, your children, your parents. These were all around me, but I could not enjoy them. All I felt was torture. This agony was blocking the enjoyment of my life. There was no real gratification out of being alive except to exist. There was only the hope that this suffering would eventually be gone. I thought it might last for a year.

This was wishful thinking as it took almost a third of my life before I felt human again!

Close to my clinic, there was an office specializing in biofeedback. If I was suffering from some sort of midlife crisis or stress problem, this treatment might help. I learned biofeedback techniques, including breathing and relaxation control. This included the exercise of tensing various parts of the body and then releasing the tension. This exercise helps a person relax and control stress. This technique had very little effect on me. I was referred to another person for hypnosis.

Lisa Painter was an accomplished hypnotist. With my biofeedback training, I seemed to do well learning self-hypnosis. During my deep hypnotic state, I felt some relief. However, once I was out of this state, my suffering continued. Lisa was especially worried about me. She was trained as a nurse. My color was very ashen and white. She checked my pulse and found it to be rapid and thready. Still, there was no explanation on what was happening to me.

I felt that every moment was my last. I had a feeling of immediate impending doom. Perhaps the most common association with this condition is an acute anxiety syndrome.

My heart seemed to quiver in my chest with a weird rhythmic vibration. The intensity and frequency of this tremor were constant. Moving around and not staying still slightly alleviated my condition. But it was not the shaking in my chest that was agonizing; it was the feeling that my body was racing a thousand miles a second without letup. The best term that I could use to describe this sensation is "morbid irritability." Everything seemed to vibrate around me. The floor was shaking, or if I leaned against a wall, the wall was shaking. The agitation that I felt was impossible to bear!

This probably does not make sense to someone who has been healthy all his life and has little awareness of poisoning. You see, mercury is neurotoxic. It kills brain cells! Picture a set of electric wires in your television: the wires are frayed and shorting out. The picture and sound become distorted and difficult to make out.

We are not just micro-circuitry. We are complex organic beings with feelings. So when there is damage to our nervous system, we can suffer a myriad of emotional and psychological symptoms. And since we live in the real world where we have to earn an income and cope in today's complex society, mercury poisoning can be an overwhelming handicap.

Imagine, if you will, not sleeping for about three years. Imagine that finally, about 7:00 a.m., you are so exhausted that you black out for a minute or two. My nights were unbelievable nightmares. They were horrible. The feeling of immediate impending death was worst at night, as if I was having a heart attack. I remember in the middle of the night occasionally feeling as though my brain was shrinking or drying out. It is hard to put this experience into words. This happened during the first year of my complete inability to perform my dental practice. I waited for the morning to come, hoping there would be some relief. Morning came, but there was no relief. The agony continued.

During a rare time that I got some sleep, I perhaps had what they call an "out of body experience." I had not experienced this before. My dream was so real, so vivid! I was flying above some local stores. I could clearly see the numbers in front of the stores. It was so real. I felt that if I could not get out of this dream, I would not be able to come back. I was alarmed by the clarity and vividness of the dream. With effort, I pulled myself out of this weird lifelike dream. I read somewhere that victims of mercury poisoning have had similar experiences.

During the night, my circulation was very bad. My arms and legs would completely go to sleep. You know the feeling you get when you sleep on an arm and you have to rub it to get the circulation back. But it was not just one arm for me. My two arms and two legs were completely asleep and had no circulation. This happened night after night. I would often rub my arms and my legs to get the circulation back. This particular problem lasted for several months.

Upon getting out of bed in the morning, my fingers would make an audible cracking sound every time I bent them. They were very stiff after not being moved during the night. This must have been an early form of arthritis induced by the mercury. In subsequent years, as I recovered, this was one of the symptoms that disappeared.

I had severe pain in various joints and muscles. After several weeks, the pain would travel to other areas. This experience just did not make sense. My symptoms numbered more than thirty.

I often had a horrible metallic taste in my mouth. I was constantly nauseous. Life was absolutely hell. Eating temporarily alleviated the nausea. However, after eating, I would feel a horror that is hard to describe. The constant morbid agitation would take on a new character. This morbid feeling was strange and hard to explain and was related to the food I was eating. Each food had its own brand of suffering for me. Although most of these food related reactions have been gone for some time now, I still suffer from a wheat allergy. These food reactions intensified my irritability. Intense attacks of irritability made it almost impossible for me to concentrate or think. My thoughts would become very scattered. It was difficult to focus on a task or carry out a project.

About noontime, I was so exhausted that my body felt as though it weighed ten tons. I had to lie down. I could hardly breathe. I could not sleep or nap. I could just endure. After about two hours, my discomfort would lessen so that I could move a bit. I would drink some water and take a vitamin C tablet, which seemed to help slightly.

Later on in the day, my cough would start. I would cough for hours without letup. Sometimes it was so severe, I could hardly catch my breath. The cough went on for almost a year. At times, I would get a strong metallic taste after coughing. All this time, the morbid agitation did not let up.

Mercury robs you of what it means to be human. It takes away your ability to have joy and really feel alive.

In my medical checkups, it was found out that my hematocrit (size and quantity of red blood cells) was high. This condition is called polycythemia. I believe that mercury can inhibit the transfer of oxygen from hemoglobin into the cells. Mercury can reduce the oxygen carrying capacity of hemoglobin. In an effort to compensate for this problem, the body may try to produce more hemoglobin which raises the hematocrit level.

After the mercury spill, one of my initial symptoms was constant diarrhea. Also strangely, my blood pressure was running slightly high.

Then, no longer was I experiencing diarrhea. Now I was constipated. At that point, all hell broke loose. I guess the diarrhea was a way for my body to rid itself of the mercury. Once I was blocked up, the mercury could no longer escape, and I started suffering the extreme ravages of mercury poisoning.

Although, at this point, I was not suspicious of mercury toxicity, I sought medical attention. I made an appointment with Dr. Birkner for the constipation problem. He is a gastroenterologist. He said that I had a common problem. He told me that I had irritable bowel syndrome and that I should take Metamucil. He found something interesting at this time, however. It did not make any sense then. He determined that I had dermatographia. This is a form of skin writing. It is one of the key identifiers of mercury poisoning, according to the World Health Organization.

The following is a statement published in a newspaper by a friend of mine:

> *"One of Dr. Scheckner's friends and patient, Ellie* of Sarasota, remarked of his behavior and physical appearance in 1989. 'As the years gradually passed,' she said, 'I began to notice a severe change (in Scheckner). His mood would change radically in a matter of hours. He seemed sometimes tired, sometimes depressed, sometimes short-tempered, sometimes angry. I wondered what was happening to this man, who had in the past enjoyed boating, family outings, and just plain having fun with his friends,' she said. 'How could this man have changed so dramatically within a matter of a couple of years?' said Ellie. 'Physically the change was, at the least, drastic! I hadn't seen Stuart in a few months, and didn't recognize him when his family came to the front door. He was so thin, he looked like a*

> *man in the final stages of the disease AIDS,' she recalled. 'As I hugged him hello, I could feel all his bones, and was certain if I had squeezed at all, he would crumble in my arms!'"*

My health continued to deteriorate, and my bizarre symptoms did not go away. Thus started my "search for health." I did not know until years later that my nemesis was mercury poisoning. In trying to find out what had happened to me, I was accused of "doctor hopping" by the opposition in my workers' compensation case.

Before my ordeal, I had a high respect for the average doctor. Now, I still respect their knowledge, but I realize their failures in handling certain medical problems are serious.

Chapter 8

First Mercury Diagnosis

I had found out about Roy Kupsinel, MD, through a newsletter that he published, "Health Consciousness". I called him on the phone and told him about my problems and made an appointment for an examination. Dr. Kupsinel's office was in Oviedo, just outside of Orlando, Florida. He recommended an exam and the mercury patch test.

Dr. Kupsinel applied a Band-Aid with mercuric chloride (.02 percent solution) to the inside of my forearm. Within two hours of this application, my arm started to burn furiously. I was outside my brother-in-law's house in Altamonte Springs (outside Orlando, Florida). I could not believe what I saw. A large amorphous dark red blotch appeared. I wanted to run into the house and grab my camera to record this bizarre happening. But I was so engrossed watching this strange creeping blob on my arm. I thought by the time I got my camera, the blob would be gone.

That night, my anxiety was extreme, which was accompanied by severe fatigue. I remember being very irritable with no patience for anything. The next morning, while I was outside in the sun, my body had red blotches all over. When Dr. Kupsinel removed the Band-Aid, there was a dark red square where the gauze had contacted my skin. It was still burning severely. Dr. Kupsinel made a diagnosis of mercury poisoning based on my symptoms and the mercury patch test.

Dr. Kupsinel told me about Rodman Shipman, MD, an orthomolecular psychiatrist. I made an appointment with Dr. Shipman, whose office was in the Orlando area. After going over my symptoms and interviewing me, he referred to a little black covered medical book and described my condition. I asked him whether the burning in my mouth was also related to mercury. He said, "Yes."

I later received a letter from Dr. Shipman. He stated that I did not need psychiatric treatment and that I had mercury poisoning. Most physicians would not have had a clue. They would have assumed the condition was all in my head, a psychiatric problem. They would have been half-right: it was mercury in my head!

Dr. Roy Kupsinel passed away from pancreatic cancer. He was a wonderful spiritual man. I would like the following to be recorded on his behalf. It was part of a deposition he gave for me in my workers' compensation proceedings. He stated this in the late 1980s, many years before the present financial fiasco and the global warming threat. I would like him to be remembered for his foresight and kindness:

> "We are undergoing a tremendous degeneration in our country. Not only physically and mentally like you're talking about concerning the medical profession, but there's a social degeneration. There's degeneration in our government. There's degeneration in the financial system of the world and there's degeneration in the planet itself, in the environment, the pollution, the air, the food and the water. And, unless people like me and others are able to raise their consciousness and bring about changes now, we will not be here tomorrow.
>
> And, one vivid example of a now is this young, wonderful person, Stuart Scheckner, who is zapped from being a dentist and serving mankind because of what he has been using has to a large degree been poisoning him."
>
> Roy Kupsinel, MD

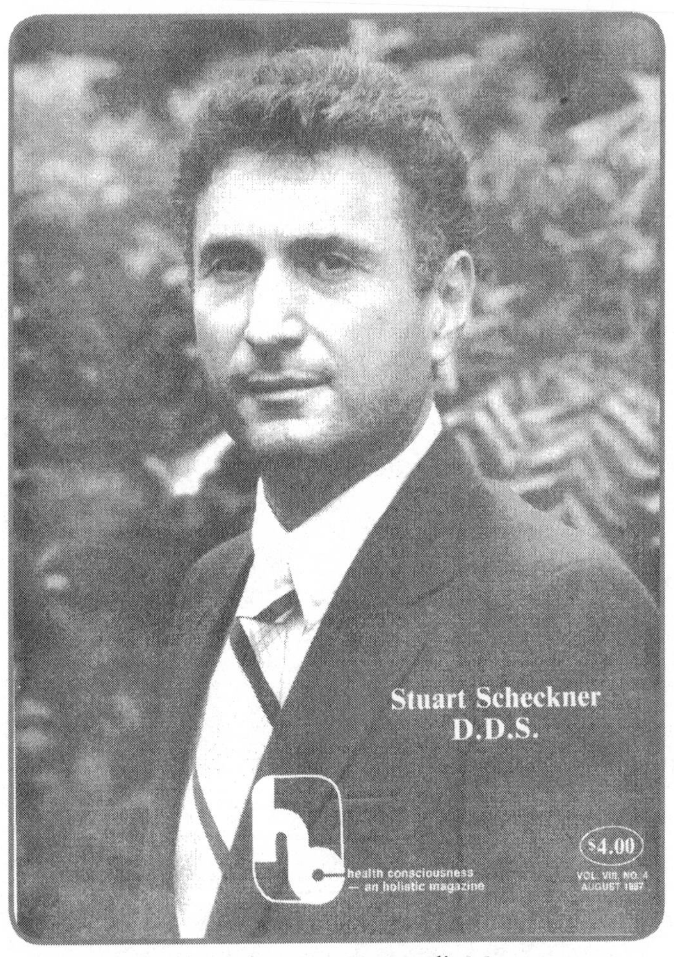

Featured article in Dr. Kupsinel's Magazine,
"Health Consciousness"
August, 1987

Chapter 9

Dr. Hal Huggins

I must give Dr. Huggins credit for saving my life. If it were not for his course that I had taken in Orlando, I probably would not have made an association between my symptoms and the mercury exposure. My name was placed on a list interested in mercury toxicity. Subsequently, I received Dr. Alfred Stock's transcript on mercury toxicity. For the first time, I became aware of the symptoms of mercury toxicity. I read Stock's description of his own mercury poisoning. Chills went through my body when I suddenly realized that the symptoms he described were happening to me!

I remember my phone call to Dr. Hal Huggins. I said to him, "I feel that I am dying, that every minute is going to be my last." I asked Dr. Huggins, "How do I get out of the woods?" The suffering was unbearable. It was a morbid agitation and a feeling of imminent death beyond any comprehension or verbal description.

Dr. Huggins recommended IV vitamin C. He was not keen on using IV EDTA for treatment. Referring to my dental amalgams, he stated, "Get that crap out of your mouth!"

I ran several hair analyses tests. My first one, with Mineral Lab, had a very high result at 18 parts per million. I called Mineral Lab and spoke to Garry F. Gordon MD, DO, PhD. Dr. Gordon said, "Thank God you found out what happened to you! Most do not." He advised me to obtain DMPS from Heyl Chemisch in Germany. At the time, DMPS was considered by some as the best chelator for mercury. A chelator is a compound that combines with metals in the treatment of metal poisoning. Today, there are better choices. I tried to obtain DMPS from Heyl Chemisch. The first time that I ordered DMPS, the FDA (Food and Drug Administration) stopped the shipment. Here I was, deathly ill and not able to get the best treatment at that time since this drug was not available in the United States.

I established a professional relationship with a new physician, Terry S. Friedmann, MD. He practiced integrative medicine. He seemed to have some knowledge of mercury. Upon the advice of Dr. Huggins, the IV vitamin C procedure was carried out.

After the IV vitamin C procedure, my symptoms that evening got much worse. Vitamin C is a weak chelator. The problem with many chelators is that they loosen mercury from one compartment of the body and then redistribute it. It is like stirring up a beehive. Sam Queen, in his book, *Chronic Mercury Toxicity*, describes the use of IV-C in detoxing mercury from the body.

I met an associate of Dr. Friedmann. He stated to me that mercury in the body is like putting "sand in a finely tuned watch." It is hard for most physicians to understand how a substance can cause so many symptoms and so much damage. Mercury has a strong affinity for sulfhydryl (SH: sulfur-hydrogen) groups in the body. The result is that so many processes of the body are affected, and then a myriad of symptoms follow. Since mercury is primarily neurotoxic and secondarily immunotoxic, the symptoms revolve mainly around these systems but not exclusively. There is so much damage that mercury can do.

At Dr. Friedmann's office, I met Dianne Ladd, a famous movie actress. Dianne is very much into holistic health care and was visiting Dr. Friedmann at the time. She was very consoling and told me to write a book about my ordeal and mention her in it. Although I was suffering at the time, she lifted my spirits. She made me feel that what happened to me would not be in vain, that I was going to make a difference in the world. It is over thirty years ago now. I hope this is the time that I would make a difference. It takes years for the truth to come out, as in the case of the tobacco- and asbestos-induced health problems. The facts are in on the dangers posed by mercury from dental amalgams or any source of mercury. Now, it is time to make the public aware of this real health problem.

After my three-day course with Dr. Huggins, I started writing articles in a local newspaper in Sarasota. The local dental board notified me to stop writing about mercury in silver fillings, or I would have to face consequences. I stopped writing because I did not want any grief. However, my dental colleague and very good friend David stopped using dental amalgam. He stood up for me at a dental board meeting when a young dentist at the board wanted to bring charges against me.

In 1987, I had a short meeting with Dr. Huggins on his visit to Sarasota. At the end of the meeting, he put his arm around me. I appreciated his friendship. The following is a letter from Dr. Huggins dated 1985. I am touched by the last paragraph in his letter:

> "I appreciate what you are doing, not just for dentistry, but in particular, for human beings. In spreading the word, making people aware is the best thing that we can do now for it takes about 4 to 5 exposures before a person really starts saying, "Yes, I have heard about that." You are good on getting that information out, and I appreciate you for that."
>
> Dr. Hal Huggins

Chapter 10

EDTA Chelation

Dr. Terry Friedmann advised me to undergo IV EDTA chelation to remove the mercury from my body. He suggested that I see Ray Evers, MD. Dr. Evers's office was in another state. Since the protocol required a series of treatments, twice a week for two months or so, it was highly impractical to obtain treatment from him.

I was very fortunate to find a local physician who performed IV EDTA therapy in Sarasota. Dr. Charles Nicholas was a DO in Sarasota. I proceeded to have the IV treatments. The therapy consisted of a slow IV drip of an EDTA preparation and lasted a couple of hours.

The nights of the first several treatments were absolutely scary. In the middle of the night, my heart would start pounding. I felt as though I was going to have a heart attack. The chelation stirs the mercury up in the body, and the symptoms are exacerbated. It was not until the tenth EDTA treatment that the reaction after the EDTA let up. I had about twenty EDTA treatments with Dr. Nicholas. The problem with mercury in the body is that as the body tries to get rid of it, it becomes reabsorbed and redistributed.

Today, there are better chelators for mercury, and these were not available when I was undergoing treatment. For instance, I met a doctor of occupational medicine. He wanted to give me BAL (British anti-lewisite or dimercaprol), which is a painful treatment and a poor choice for mercury chelation.

While I was having the chelation therapy, Donald, another patient of Dr. Nicholas's, approached me. He said, "Dr. Scheckner, I have symptoms very much like yours." We had a discussion on the mercury problems from dental fillings. Donald had a mouthful of dental amalgams and decided to have them removed. I did not discuss any protocol with him, such as precautions on removal or supplementation to aid in detoxification pathways. As I understand it, he went to a dentist who had no knowledge of the dangers of removing dental amalgams from a person who is mercury toxic. The amalgam dust created by removing mercury-silver fillings with a high speed handpiece subjected Donald to a great deal of mercury. In addition, his body's detoxification pathways were inadequate.

After the removal of his dental amalgams, he approached me. He said that he wished he never had his dental amalgams removed. He felt worse than ever! I suggested that he see a physician friend of mine whose clinic was next to my former dental office.

I had once reviewed my diary, and on an entry dated February 15, 1987, I wrote something that Donald told me that gave me the chills. In his church, the minister told the congregation the following: Eight years ago, a man who was in the back of the church asked to come forward and be baptized. He was emaciated and extremely ill. The man said to the minister, "Don't you know me?" He told the minister his name. He was a dentist, and he said he had mercury poisoning. A month later, this dentist died!

Chapter 11

Reaching Out

The entire ordeal that I went through because of my illness needed meaning. This was one of the ways for me to hold on and survive. What could I do to help other people so that my suffering would not be in vain?

The torture, minute by minute, was indescribable. Now that I am writing about it, words cannot, in any measure, capture the agony. You could look at a person whose brain is being fried and he would probably look normal. You could not tell the agony he is going through. What you would probably say is that he or she has a serious problem. You would likely say he or she has a mental problem. But what if that problem is being caused by a poisonous material that attacks the brain?

Take, for example, the Gulf War syndrome. It has taken some time to recognize that our soldiers were exposed to poisonous gases. In the beginning, all they tried to say was that it was a psychological condition caused by the stresses of the war: post-traumatic stress disorder. Now we are more aware that their condition could be due to many factors. Our soldiers were given a myriad of immunization and protective injections on a mass scale. They probably contained thimerosal, a mercury preservative. Our boys were exposed to heavy vapors of diesel fuel and other chemicals. Saddam Hussein had many chemical bunkers. We really don't know what or how many chemicals they were exposed to and how these chemicals react with each other.

It is indeed frustrating to try to obtain help for a condition that you cannot even see. For example, AIDS patients completely lose their immune system and die. That's dramatic. People stand up and pay attention. They are petrified with their thoughts that they might be exposed to such a horrible disease. But what we are talking about here is a health problem that has not much obvious impact, but it is a problem affecting all of us. We acquiesce to placing poison in our mouths under the guise of a silver filling. This silver filling is actually a mercury filling. This mercury constantly leaks into our mouths over a period of many years and slowly accumulates in our bodies. Because there is no simple test for subacute chronic mercury poisoning, it is easy to overlook the dangers that mercury poses to our health. However, the issue of mercury poisoning from dental fillings is also symbolic of what we are doing to ourselves. We drink water full of chemicals, we eat food that has been adulterated and processed, and we breathe air that is contaminated with all kinds of poisons. Never in the history of man have we been exposed to such a chemical onslaught.

The effects of all this exposure to poisons are the many degenerative diseases that afflict people. Chronic health problems appear. Physicians confronted with many maladies, whether they are organic or psychological, use medications to cover up the problem. Aspirin, Advil, ibuprofen, Tylenol, Valium, Xanax, and so on. We have all kinds of chemicals to cover up the other chemicals that our body cannot cope with anymore. With the additional onslaught on the body's detoxification system, it is no wonder why many people have certain types of medical problems. Most of the time, physicians are treating symptoms rather than getting to the causes, which are the poisons.

The medical school curriculum is so complex. There is not enough time to study preventive medicine. Medicine today is engrossed with medications and surgery. We practice emergency medicine, not preventive medicine.

A physician is the mainstay of health care. However, many people today are dissatisfied with our health care system, so they seek alternative medicine. In order to cope with our toxic environment and the stress in our daily lives, we need to enhance our body's defenses. Chemicals will not do this. We need to enrich our nutrition. We need to take biologically compatible nutrients so that we can deal with our environment. If we don't, we will suffer a long-range consequence called metabolic genocide, according to a renowned nutritionist, Henry Osiecki, from Australia.

My plea is for our country and the world to wake up before it is too late. This is my prime motivation in writing this book. We need to stop poisoning ourselves.

The following newspaper article was one of my attempts to make my message known (*Volusia Conservation Digest*, volume 1, issue 3, January 1991, Ormond Beach, Florida).

"Danger to Dentists

> *Stuart Scheckner had been practicing dentistry for 14 years in 1978. One day when he was working on a patient, an assistant spilled a bottle of mercury onto the shag rug that covered his office floor. "It fell into the carpet one foot from my chair," he said.*
>
> *Not long after the accident, he began experiencing digestive problems, and then chronic diarrhea, both poisoning symptoms. In 1979, he consulted a doctor about the symptoms and queried him about a tie-in to the spill or possible mercury poisoning. The doctor shrugged it off saying, "Forget about it. Just stay away from it." Now Scheckner wishes he had known enough to demand a urine mercury test.*
>
> *Other dentists Scheckner knows have symptoms they don't want to acknowledge; he said he has observed the telltale tremors in their hands.*
>
> *"Mercury is an extremely insidious poison, whether to dentists or patients; it's very, very difficult to diagnose," Scheckner*

explained. He compared the type of poisoning to throwing sand into a finely tuned instrument. "It fouls up the works," he said. "The mercury damages both the central nervous system and the immune system."

Scheckner, who eventually was diagnosed as having mercurial encephalopathy or abnormal brain waves, explained that mercury poisoning can closely mimic multiple sclerosis, kidney disease, digestive disturbances and respiratory disorders.

His doctor, Sandra Denton, MD, of Anchorage, Alaska, an international lecturer on mercury amalgam toxicity, says, "Ninety-five percent of medical doctors do not understand the problems and dangers of heavy metal toxicity."

But Scheckner has learned of these problems and dangers, and he wants others to know too. "There is a desperate need for the public to pressure legislators to look at the amalgam challenge, investigate the issue, and fund additional research. When we can succeed with this, maybe it will be the start of a whole new environmental age," Scheckner said."

I once met a dentist at Siesta Key Beach who had symptoms consistent with mercury poisoning. His dental office was located about a half hour away. He told me that his copying machine kept breaking down and that he was told by a technician who was trying to fix it that mercury vapor could cause such a problem. After telling this dentist that his symptoms could be related to mercury exposure, he seemed to be in denial. I imagine that many other dentists with insidious slight symptoms of mercury poisoning would feel the same way.

The following is a quote from Dr. Garry Gordon's Internet site (http://www.gordonresearch.com/factforum/welcome.html):

"As you might expect, dentists and dental assistants have a high level of exposure, although they have become much more careful in the past few years. Nonetheless, a large study of several hundred dentists and dental assistants in Washington State found that almost all of them had four or more symptoms consistent with mercury toxicity."

Chapter 12

The MS Connection

In my reading about mercury, there was a discussion on the connection of multiple sclerosis to mercury-silver fillings. My wife found the phone number of the local MS society. I made arrangements to meet Betty*, the head of the local MS society. She had a guest with her, Vivian*.

Vivian told me her amazing story. She had MS for years and her condition had been deteriorating. The priest was in her home and saying last rights for her. She had a premonition that she needed to have her mercury-silver fillings removed. She flew back up north to her dentist there. All her dental amalgams were removed. Within a few weeks, she was completely free of the MS symptoms. It was only when she would go to a beauty parlor or be exposed to some chemical that some slight symptoms would return.

My wife and I became good friends with Vivian and her husband, Al*. Vivian was a tough gal. She had been through a lot. She had suffered for years, yet she had maintained a strong, positive attitude.

In chapter 10, I referred to Donald who had his mercury fillings removed and had a severe reaction requiring medical attention. I later found out that he had been committed to the psychiatric unit at

Sarasota Memorial Hospital. I was shocked that he was there. This is the worst thing you can do to someone with mercury toxicity. They were medicating him with psychotherapeutic drugs. His reaction was so severe that he had to be placed in a straight jacket. My former physician, Dr. James, wanted me to go to the hospital obviously for psychiatric treatment. I did not go because I knew that they had no protocol for treating mercury toxicity. They would have ruined me as they did poor Donald.

I spoke to a knowledgeable psychiatrist a number of years later about the use of psychotherapeutic drugs on a mercury toxic patient. He told me that psychotherapeutic medication has an adverse effect on a mercury toxic patient. It can increase the toxicity in the patient.

I was discussing what had happened to Donald with Vivian. Vivian was good friends with Dr. Vladimir*, a psychiatrist. She told Dr. Vladimir about Donald. Donald was taken off medication. He no longer needed a straight jacket, and he was released from the hospital.

The incident with Donald occurred twenty-five years ago. I was wondering what happened to him. I was able to locate him through an Internet search. He is in a nursing home and now has Parkinson's disease. It is likely that his mercury exposure led to the onset of this disease.

In my search for a connection between mercury-silver fillings and their adverse health effects, I found out about Barbara*. What makes this such a powerful story is that the ADA stated that there has never been any harm caused by mercury-silver fillings.

Barbara had been to a medical doctor. The doctor's assistant applied a diathermy (heat-producing) machine over her jaw area. After the treatment, she did not feel well. The very next day, she had difficulty walking and had a strong metallic taste in her mouth. She told me she had brain fog. The diathermy machine had evidently heated up her dental fillings and increased the vaporization of mercury. The heat from the diathermy machine had been so intense that it had burned her gums, which had turned white. Mercury ordinarily comes off mercury-silver fillings at a very low level. A higher temperature increases this vaporization. Her four fillings had released a large amount of mercury because of the heat. Her exposure to this mercury caused neurological damage. This incident occurred in 1984 and she is still suffering its effects today.

In a letter that I read from Dr. Huggins to Barbara, Huggins said that the number of people suffering from mercury poisoning from amalgam is staggering, so what I have personally seen is just the tip of the iceberg.

Barbara introduced me to Michael McCann, MD, a pediatric immunologist. At the time, Dr. McCann was on a fellowship at All Children's' Hospital in St. Petersburg, Florida.

I made an appointment to see Dr. McCann at the hospital for my condition. Robert Good, MD, PhD, DSc, FACP, was chief of medicine at this hospital. He is the "father of modern immunology and cellular engineering."

Dr. Good came in to see me during the exam. I was very happy to meet him, a renowned physician. I talked to him about the relationship of mercury and autoimmune diseases.

Dr. Michael McCann and I became good friends. We co-authored an article in the *Journal of Clinical Pharmacy.* He felt that it would go down in the annals of medicine as a very important document. Basically, the article substantiates that mercury can act as a trigger for autoimmune diseases.

The following is a quote from an abstract that Dr. McCann and I authored:

> *"Mercury exposure should be considered for more than its classic toxicological effects. Even minuscule amounts of a foreign antigen or hapten, such as mercury, can have profound clinical effects in genetically susceptible individuals. The link between autoimmune disorders, such as thyroid dysfunction, and mercury should prove to be an important and a fertile topic of investigation".*[10]

---

10 Michael McCann and Stuart Scheckner, "Hyperthyroidism Associated with Mercury Poisoning," *Journal of Clinical Pharmacy* 10 (1991): 742–743.

Chapter 13

The Basophilic Degranulation Study

While I was a patient of Dr. Terry Friedmann, I contacted a lab on the east coast of Florida. I spoke to Frank*, PhD, an immunologist. I explained my problem to him, and he agreed to see me. I made an appointment and met with Dr. Frank in his office.

Since I lived on the west coast of Florida, I had to drive across the state. I arrived at Dr. Frank's office late in the afternoon. He took a sample of my blood and looked at it under one of his high-tech microscopes. He said that there was no evidence of mercury in my blood. It was kind of frustrating that I could not find the cause of my problems. However, I was aware that mercury in the blood is only present for a short amount of time after exposure. I wondered if Dr. Frank was aware of that. Anyway, he told me to come back in the morning.

Dr. Frank took another sample of my blood in the morning and placed it under another large microscope. As he was examining the blood slide, he seemed excited and called me over to take a look. He said that the large colorful flower-like structures were memory cells. He explained to me that in order for my body to produce these memory cells, my immune system had to have undergone an extreme challenge. I asked him if my prolonged exposure to mercury could have caused the production these cells. He replied in the affirmative. Perhaps these memory cells had made me so highly reactive to the mercury exposure in my last six months of dental practice.

Dr. Frank took me to an Indian restaurant. I had never been to an Indian restaurant before and enjoyed the experience of having a dish with curry seasoning. We discussed the prospects of developing a test for mercury. He said that he could do it. I was impressed that Dr. Frank could do research and create a testing protocol.

After some time, Dr. Frank notified me that he was ready to do the project. The test he created for the mercury study was called the "basophilic degranulation test." We were going to run a type of double-blind study. He obtained a sample of blood from a control. The results on the control were negative. If we obtained a positive reaction from a patient, therefore, it would be significant.

I talked to my physician, Dr. Friedmann, about obtaining volunteers for this study. He was agreeable and found patients who had multiple nonspecific symptoms that were hard to explain. Finding these people did not seem a difficult task for Dr. Friedmann. In an average practice, it would probably not be too hard to find patients with this type of profile. These patients would normally be written off as having mental or some other problems and medicated. I had eleven volunteers and myself, making a total of twelve subjects. A special mercury medical questionnaire was completed by all patients. The complaints listed by the patients were numerous. This medical questionnaire by Dr. Huggins is in the appendix of this book.

Barbara was part of the group. She had been exposed to an excessive amount of mercury from her fillings through the application of a diathermy machine over her facial area. Her test came out positive for mercury.

The results on Mrs. Kathryn* were negative for mercury but positive for nickel. This was very compelling. Kathryn had no mercury-silver fillings in her mouth. Instead, she had many nickel crowns in her mouth. We had a discussion about having her nickel crowns removed and replaced with noble metals (gold alloy). Sometime later, she told me that her nickel crowns had been removed. She felt much better, and her medical complaints were gone!

When you look at the medical questionnaire, you will see multiple symptoms that do not seem to have a relationship. When there is a condition where there are many symptoms that do not seem related, then one needs to look into the possibility of a systemic poison that is affecting overall health. Mercury is such a poison especially affecting the nervous and immune systems.

Results of test: Ten of the twelve subjects were positive for mercury in the basophilic degranulation test. Considering that the control sample was negative, this is highly suggestive of a relationship between exposure to mercury and a low-grade toxic effect.

Would it not be prudent for a physician to be aware that a patient with diverse medical complaints may have a systemic toxicity problem? Every general practitioner, every cardiologist, every neurologist, every psychiatrist, every psychologist, every endocrinologist, every pulmonologist, every urologist, every ob-gyn, and every ENT specialist should have a copy of a similar health questionnaire. When a patient presents multisystem complaints with a psychological overtone, you need to be suspicious of a systemic poison, especially mercury. It is not a psychiatric problem. It is an organic toxicological problem!

I made an appointment with Dr. Ron*, a neurologist. I handed him a printed list of my symptoms. As he read it, he nodded his head as if he understood my problem. He said, "You have *temporal lobe dysfunction*." He was the first doctor to diagnose temporal lobe dysfunction (encephalopathy or abnormal brain function) in me. Yet when I asked him whether mercury exposure could have caused this problem, he said, "Yes, but what is a dentist doing with mercury?" I believe that many other good physicians would answer the same way. Obviously, if a physician is not aware that mercury is used in dental practice, it is unlikely that he would be aware that the dentist and his patients are exposed to mercury.

Dr. Ron sent me for an EEG (electroencephalogram). The outcome was abnormal. The test involves attaching electric leads to your scalp. A reading is taken to show whether the electrical brain activity is normal. The results gave an abnormal reading. I had encephalopathy.

Subsequently, he sent me for a specific test for temporal lobe dysfunction. In this test, in addition to the wire leads on the scalp, the technician placed wire leads up both of my nostrils into my sinus. It was a very uncomfortable procedure, first, to get the leads through my nostrils, and second, into my sinuses. I remember the technician had a great deal of difficulty removing these wire leads, and I was extremely uncomfortable as these leads were stuck in my nostrils and my sinuses.

The diagnosis of temporal lobe dysfunction was confirmed by this test. The temporal lobe is one of the basic subdivisions of the brain. There is one temporal lobe on the right side and one on the left side of the brain.

Chapter 14

Mis-Education from the American Dental Association

The ADA has various publications on mercury hygiene. As I went through the journals and literature from the American Dental Association, I found various warnings about the storage of amalgam scrap. Amalgam scrap is the leftover amalgam from carving a restoration and the excess not used. This has to be stored in a closed jar to contain the mercury vapor. (The dental patient must ask, "How can this be safe in my mouth at 98.6 degrees Fahrenheit and not be safe out of the mouth at room temperature?")

In addition, at a number of dental conventions, there were mercury tests available. Urine mercury levels of dentists were tested for exposure.

I contacted the ADA for help. Surely, they would be able to assist me with their knowledge. I wrote them a letter, giving them information about my problem. I also gave them my urine mercury level. The diagnosis of low-level mercury toxicity is extremely complex. The response letter I got from the ADA was a mixture of fact and contradiction to much of the scientific peer review on the subject. I believe Dr. Lane* meant well. Sadly, his letter would have severely misled me. This is, however, the classical conventional thinking of many in medicine today. (References made to the ADA are from Dr. Lane's letter to me.)

Whether you are a dentist or a dental patient, you face the same problem with regard to the diagnosis of mercury toxicity. For the dental patient reading this book, please put yourself in my shoes. You are in the same boat as I am with regard to the diagnosis of mercury toxicity, you from your mercury-silver fillings and me from occupational exposure to mercury. Mercury is recognized as an occupational hazard in dentistry but not a hazard caused by mercury-silver fillings. If you have multiple unrelated symptoms, such as those in the medical questionnaire found in the appendix of this book, and suspect a mercury problem, your physician might run a urine mercury test. It is probable that, despite a mouthful of mercury-silver fillings and symptoms, your urine mercury level is below average. This is likely a sign of "mercury retention"; your kidneys are losing their ability to excrete mercury. If your physician is unaware of how mercury retention problems occur, he might wrongly interpret the low level of urinary mercury as indicating that the problem is not caused by mercury. Your physician would then rule out mercury poisoning.

One must understand the significance of urine mercury levels. On a group basis, they are significant as they reveal the exposure of a large group of people. However, on an individual basis, they are not significant. The ADA is making a false assertion that on an individual basis, urine mercury levels must be high to make a diagnosis of toxicity. Dr. Lane of the ADA states thus: "Your urinary mercury levels are well within the normal range of the general asymptomatic population. In fact, your levels of urinary mercury are *less* than the mean urinary mercury levels of dentists surveyed from 1975–1983 in the Association's Health Assessment program which was 14.2 µgHg/l [micrograms of mercury per liter]." Dentists as a group have mean urine mercury levels that are above the average population, so these do work in group studies.

The ADA is saying that my urine mercury levels are less than the average dentist's, and therefore, I have no mercury-induced problem. This is wrong information, mis-education. Well, how does that explain how my urine mercury levels are so low that they are undetectable? My hair analyses from *two* different laboratories, however, came back as high toxic levels. The ADA excludes the use of hair analysis in making a diagnosis of mercury toxicity since the mercury could have come from the air. But you need some logic here. I had not gone to my dental office for quite a few months, so there was no external exposure to mercury. This mercury in my hair, therefore, was coming from within my body. How could I have high mercury in my hair and yet no mercury in my urine? The ADA's teaching about urine mercury testing does not make sense. Regarding hair analysis, sometimes very mercury toxic people have low levels of mercury in their hair also. What is coming out of the body is not necessarily what is in the body!

With regard to the validity of using hair analysis for detecting heavy metals, Dale Jenkins did a hair analysis study for the EPA (Environmental Protection Agency) on the Minamata Bay disaster (Japan, 1932–1968). I met with Dale Jenkins in Sarasota to discuss his research for the EPA. A factory dumped mercury into the Minamata Bay and contaminated the fish. "Over 3,000 victims have been recognized as having 'Minamata Disease.' People consumed the fish which caused many deaths and abnormalities. Many people have lost their lives, suffered from physical deformities, or have had to live with the physical and emotional pain of 'Minamata Disease.'"

The point is that the EPA used hair analysis to determine levels of toxicity. Hair analysis, therefore, is a valid tool in analyzing heavy metals, however, with limitations. The hair analysis study shows a temporal relationship. If mercury or a heavy metal does not show in the hair, it does not exclude a body burden of the heavy metal. Some of the sickest, most mercury-poisoned people have *low* levels of mercury in their hair. Such people have lost their ability to excrete mercury through their hair.

My urine mercury level was undetectable. With regard to using it to rule out mercury as my problem, Dr. Lane, of the ADA, made the following statement: "However, the lowest levels at which symptoms of mercury toxicity have been reported are from 150 μgHg/l to 200 μgHg/l."

Dr. Lane is contradicting documentation from our own *Journal of the American Dental Association* (*JADA*):

> "Acute symptoms generally follow a long-term exposure because the individual becomes sensitized. Urinalysis tests for mercury are reliable for screening evaluations to discover exposure, but because the urinary mercury level drops with the onset of symptoms of mercurial poisoning, this test is not dependable to determine toxic reaction."[11]

In addition, the following highly credible citation from the National Institute for Occupational Safety and Health contradicts Dr. Lane's contention that you have to have high mercury levels in urine to have mercury poisoning:

> "There is no "critical" level of mercury in urine above or below which poisoning cannot be seen."[12]

Other studies show that urine mercury levels do *not* correlate with mercury exposure, such as the following:

> "Concentration of mercury in the urine, blood, and hair . . , assumption, even if it is generally accurate, is not sufficiently effective in daily clinical diagnosis because there is great individual variation with regard to susceptibility to mercury.
>
> Studies failed to find the characteristic signs and symptoms of poisoning as a result of overexposure. This was in spite of the fact that mercury levels in the workers' urine were high (sometimes reaching 500μg/l).
>
> Clear, negative and significant correlation was found between time on the job and the level of mercury in the urine. In other words, the longer a worker is on the job, the less mercury is excreted in his urine.
>
> Since this measure (urine) indicates the efficiency with which the kidneys flush out mercury and not necessarily

---

11 N. W. Rupp and G. C. Paffenbarger, "Reports of Councils and Bureaus, Significance to Health of Mercury Used in Dental Practice: A Review," *JADA* 82 (June 1971): 1406.

12 National Institute for Occupational Safety and Health.

> the level of mercury in the body or blood, it can be used neither as a reliable measure of subclinical damage nor as a correlate of such a measure."[13]

The above reference indicates that urine mercury levels decreased with time since the body had become *less* efficient in removing mercury, not because the workers had become less mercury poisoned.

The American Dental Association, at the end of the letter, stated, "Please do not let the unproven theories of retention-toxicity distract you from seeking the primary cause and appropriate treatment of your illness". The latest science contradicts the ADA's position. The fact is that urine mercury levels do *not* show the body burden of mercury; they only indicate the mercury coming out in the urine.

The ADA asserted that my symptoms suggested I had Graves' disease. They ruled out mercury toxicity because of my low or nonexistent urine mercury levels. I thought the same. I expected that when my T4 (thyroxin) levels became normal through treatment, I would be cured and feel better. Instead, my symptoms got worse. My thyroid disease was a result of mercury exposure, not the cause of my illness.

It has been documented by Trakhtenberg, a Russian scientist, that mercury exposure can trigger Graves' disease in occupationally mercury-exposed workers. Again, the ADA misled me on the subject. The ADA makes statements from a position of authority but not from a position of the scientific facts. My case is proof of that.[14]

The American Dental Association has been using erroneous criteria to assert that mercury-silver fillings are safe. Low urine mercury levels are used to rule out mercury toxicity in individuals who have symptoms of poisoning. This is a standard that most physicians use. Mercury

---

13 O. Lamm and H. Pratt, "Sub-Clinical Effects of Exposure to Inorganic Mercury Revealed Somatosensory-Evoked Potentials," *Eur Neurol* 24 (1985): 237–243.

14 Michael McCann and Stuart Scheckner, "Hyperthyroidism Associated with Mercury Poisoning," *Journal of Clinical Pharmacy* 10 (1991): 742–743.

is extremely insidious since it is so hard to diagnose. To make things worse, it is the most potent neurotoxic non-radioactive element on earth.

Although the information Dr. Lane provided me was misguided, I appreciate his attempt to assist me.

Chapter 15

American Biologics Hospital

I was desperate. I thought every minute was going to be my last.

While I was reviewing my diary, I noticed a varied progression. I had some days that I felt better, some days that the cough let up, some days of muscle and joint pain, etc. The constant nausea was horrible after I would eat. I remember taking licorice powder to help soothe my stomach and alleviate the nausea.

An excerpt from my diary dated 1986:

> "It is hard to point all the ideas and thoughts down. The effect and affect on one's mind, the anxiety, the irritability, the emotions, the feelings that change due to varying effects of toxicity. For instance, yesterday I went for acupuncture. This was the second time I had gone to St. Petersburg to Dr. Y. Immediately after treatment, I was pleasantly relaxed. In the evening, we went to a show. During this time, I felt fatigued and uneasy. I had a feeling of a buzz in my chest. It was disconcerting.
>
> I remember the phone call from Fred Engelmann. He said he died a thousand deaths already. Fred wrote a book

> on mercury from silver fillings. Fred included me in his book: *The Iatrogenesis Factor: A Quicksilver Mystery*, F. C. Engelmann.
>
> It is the constant unrelenting suffering that wears you down. Not being able to enjoy your family, your children, and your own life."

When I read the above diary entry, words cannot express the torture. Only by going through the suffering can one understand this unbelievable agony. Another mercury toxic dentist, Dr. Greg*, said to me, "I would not wish this on my worst enemy!" There are several other mercury toxic dentists whom I had contacted through the years, and they had almost the same symptoms.

I was desperate. The suffering was unbearable. Somehow, I came across a clinic in Mexico that treated mercury toxicity.

On October 13, 1986, I left for the American Biologics Hospital in Tijuana, Mexico. They said they treat industrial poisoning and Candida. In many cases of mercury toxicity, there is a problem with opportunistic organisms such as *Candida albicans*. It becomes a systemic problem when the immune system is compromised, such as in AIDS and mercury toxicity. The treatment at the American Biologics consisted of IV EDTA, dioxychlor, vitamins, gerivitol, and live cell injections. I was not all too sure of the benefits and the risks of this treatment, but I had to try it. Doing nothing was not an option.

While I was at the American Biologics Hospital, I talked to Dr. Kuhnau, an immunologist. I asked him whether there was a relationship between mercury toxicity and hyperthyroidism. He affirmed that my hyperthyroidism was the result of mercury intoxication.

On January 9, 1987, I received a call from Dr. Tapia, one of my physicians at the American Biologics Hospital. He said the live cell therapy should have some effects around this time. I told him that there had been some days without tremors. Perhaps this was a sign that I was on my way to recovery. However, this did not happen dramatically. My suffering went on for many years. There were periods of less agony. I had many symptoms, and they would come and go. I had arthritis-like symptoms in my hands. Pain in my joints was not uncommon. Upon waking up in the morning, my fingers made a cracking sound when I tried to move them.

Also, if you think you have a mercury-related problem, your doctor might order a urine mercury and/or blood mercury test. Since the doctor does not know how to diagnose low-level subacute mercury toxicity, you might be misled by negative findings. We are dealing with one of the most insidious neurotoxic materials known to man, and most mainstream health professionals lack knowledge in this field.

So with all this *ignorance*, I was led into a trap:

I carried medical insurance through my dental practice. When I submitted my medical charges from the American Biologics Hospital, the insurance carrier paid their share of the bill. However, they told me they would no longer cover my medical expenses because I had a work-related medical problem. They told me to apply for workers' compensation to pay my medical bills. If I knew then what I know now, I would have never done it. Workers' compensation turned out to be an ordeal of time, stress, humiliation, and money that I could not afford. What did they use against me? *Ignorance* and more!

ABC Insurance Company* was my medical insurance carrier for my office. They had paid part of my medical bills from Dr. Charles Nicholas and the American Biologics Hospital. They sent me a letter that they were discontinuing my medical coverage since my problem was work related. They told me to apply for workers' compensation.

Chapter 16

My Workers' Compensation Case

I looked through the yellow pages under the workers' compensation lawyers category and found Attorney Douglas*. I met with him, and he seemed to take an interest in my case. He indicated that I had a fair chance of winning.

I had workers' compensation insurance under my dental corporation. Attorney Kyle* was the local attorney of the insurance company. Prior to giving an initial deposition to Attorney Kyle, I met with Attorney Douglas. I asked Attorney Douglas whether I should mention the spill of mercury in my shag carpeting. The spill occurred in 1978, and it was now 1987. Although I only found out recently that I had mercury poisoning, he suggested that I should not mention the spill since it might create a problem with the statute of limitations. When the spill was made known at a later date, Attorney Kyle claimed that we had changed the case.

When I had retained Attorney Douglas, I did not know that he had taken over Attorney Andy's* law practice. Attorney Andy was on leave. When Attorney Andy returned to his practice, he took over my case. I heard that the hearing officer, the judge, for Sarasota, and Attorney

Andy were not the best of friends. I did not feel too good about this situation since my case could have many obstacles.

I felt that it was important for me to find Linda, the secretary who spilled mercury. I tried to find Linda but could not.

We had been to a wedding one time with Linda. At the wedding, we were introduced to Attorney Jason*. I was able to locate Jason and asked him if he could contact Linda for me. I believe that he was able to contact Linda's mother to find out where Linda was. He finally contacted Linda and asked her about the spill. She said that she could not remember the spill. She was not a trained assistant and had no idea of the danger of a mercury spill. When she spilled the mercury, to her, it was no more dangerous than spilling water. Therefore, she could not remember the incident.

If I had only reprimanded Linda for spilling the mercury, then she would have remembered! I was too busy and under too much pressure since my dental assistant was out. I guess, in life, there are things that you regret not doing because you later know it would have made a difference.

I told Attorney Jason what had happened and informed him that I had been advised by my medical insurance carrier to file a workers' compensation case.

Attorney Jason was intrigued by my case. He had an interest in the medical aspects of it. He agreed to take on my case but said he would have to brush up on workers' compensation law.

After some time, Jason said that he could only cover the merits of the case, the medical part, and that Attorney Andy would have to cover the legal procedural part.

Jason had me do a project:

1. Medical records of all physicians seen
2. Peer review medical abstracts related to mercury poisoning with symptoms

3. Annotated and collated medical records with peer review medical literature on mercury poisoning

Reviewing it now, I am amazed by this documented study on a case of mercury toxicity—me! I learned a great deal on the subject of mercury toxicity doing this report. The first two parts of the project filled two large loose-leaf books. The third part was a report collating all the information in those documents with annotations relating both my medical history and peer review medical reports. It was 31 pages long.

I remember one time sitting down with Attorney Jason and having a conversation about my case. He had heard that the insurance company had told their lawyer, Attorney Kyle, to spare no expense in winning the case against me.

My case was going extremely slow. It had been continued numerous times, and the judge could not seem to wait to get it off his books. I could not do more than I was doing. I was trying to get documentation on my case. It was not easy. I found Dr. M* in Tampa, who specialized in occupational medicine. He seemed clueless about my diagnosis of mercury toxicity since my urine mercury levels were undetectable, below an average non-exposed person's.

I had an appointment with Dr. Nicholas Alexiou at the University of South Florida's College of Medicine. Dr. Alexiou is a specialist in occupational medicine. This was his statement: "Impression: History of mercury exposure and sensitization with a secondary anxiety reaction and increased stress response. No explanation for other than the possibility of mercury poisoning for multiple symptoms."

Dr. Alexiou's statement was quite accurate. However, it was not strong enough to settle the adversarial legal problems in dealing with the judge and the defense legal counsel, Kyle.

I had seen several physicians for mercury toxicity at this point.

Dr. Roy Kupsinel's diagnosis was mercury toxicity. He had performed the mercuric chloride patch test on me, and the results showed that I was highly sensitive to mercury.

Dr. Rodman Shipman, an orthomolecular psychiatrist, had told me, "Dr. Scheckner, you do not need psychoanalysis. You have mercury poisoning!"

Dr. Leonard Haimes had been seeing me for my mercury toxicity. His medical office was on the east coast of Florida, across the state from me. He helped me get off the Inderal, which was controlling my tachycardia (fast heart rate).

I had heard about Sandra Denton, MD, who specialized in mercury toxicity. I made an appointment to see her in Kent, Washington. She stated in her medical report on me: "His symptoms were classic for mercury toxicity." I spent a full week being tested at her office. The testing was very extensive. At the time, she was associated with Dr. Jonathan Wright. Dr. Wright is a leader in alternative medicine. Since I knew about him, I wanted to meet him, and I spent a few minutes talking to him.

Dr. Denton suggested that I contact Louis Chang, PhD, since he was one of the leading experts in mercury toxicology. I contacted Dr. Chang, and he agreed to be my expert witness. He complimented me for standing up for my rights.

Serious Breach of Confidentiality

Dr. Shield* was retained by the defense attorney, Attorney Kyle, to evaluate my case. He had in his possession a copy of the letter that Dr. Lane sent me on behalf of the American Dental Association (ADA) stating that I did not have mercury toxicity. His evaluation, with the support of the letter from Dr. Lane, was used to show that I did not have mercury toxicity. The correspondence between Dr. Lane of the ADA and me was a privileged communication and contained confidential information. When I saw this breach of confidentiality, I sent a letter to the ADA. The following letter, dated June 20, 1990, is the reply from the ADA legal department:

> "Dear Dr. Scheckner:
>
> Thank you for your letter of May 4, regarding your workers' compensation case . . .

> Have investigated your concern that confidentiality have been breached and can now assure you they have not. Dr. Lane indicated he did not send the letter to Dr. Shield. Dr. Shield indicated he received all material in connection with your case from the attorneys.
>
> Is it possible, Dr. Scheckner, that the letter was produced in the workers' compensation case as a part of routine discovery? In the usual course of litigation, such information would be discoverable by the opposing party, absent some privilege."

I did not give Dr. Lane's letter to my attorneys. At the time, I would have remembered it if I did and would have contacted my attorneys regarding this matter instead of the ADA. So how did this letter appear? Dr. Shield claimed that he received it from the defense attorneys. Defense Attorney Kyle would not even had known that this letter from the A.D.A. existed since I was the only recipient of this letter.

Now, here is the big question. If the above is correct, then how did the defense attorney, Kyle, acquire this privileged confidential letter? There is a serious breach of confidentiality. The mystery is who is responsible. Who had access to this letter from the ADA?

This erroneous information from the ADA was incorporated into documents in my workers' compensation case. Instead of supporting me by providing correct information, my own American Dental Association gave misleading information that hurt me. Louis Chang, PhD, one of the foremost mercury toxicologists in the world, was an expert witness on my side. The A.D.A., therefore, was in direct contradiction with one of the leading scientists in the world on my case.

The Day Before The Final Hearing

The day of the final hearing was fast approaching. The judge had warned that he would not allow any more delays.

Dr. Chang had sent me a letter indicating that he was concerned. No one had contacted him to make arrangements for the final hearing. He was ready. He warned me that time was running out.

Dr. Sandra Denton had performed an extensive one-week testing program in Kent, Washington, to determine my medical condition. Her diagnosis was that I had "classic mercury toxicity." I had sent her letters requesting a medical report on my diagnosis and condition. She was very busy with her medical practice, and it was difficult for her to spend time to write the report. This report required much of her time because the issue was complex. I took the blame for not getting this report, but there was little I could do. Attorney Andy, the lawyer who was handling the legal procedural aspects of my case, notified me several times that I needed this report for my case.

Prior to the final hearing, we were to have Dr. Sandra Denton give a deposition. She was to give a one-on-one personal report to both the defense attorney and my attorney. Since Attorney Jason was handling the merits of my case, he would fly to Colorado for the deposition. The defense attorney's office objected. They said they were not given adequate time to make arrangements to depose Dr. Denton in Colorado. This objection was agreed to by the judge. The defense did not have to go to Colorado. At the same time, the defense attorney objected to a phone deposition. The phone is commonly used for depositions, especially when distance is involved. The defense attorney was not going to allow this equitable request.

The day before the final hearing, my legal procedural counsel, Attorney Andy, was in Colorado. I was apprehensive about what was happening. A phone call to Attorney Andy's office was not enough at this point. I went to his office to find out what was going on. After several hours of waiting, Carol*, his paralegal, assured me that everything was okay. She would have the case continued. She would schedule a new final hearing to allow us to continue the case.

I called my merits Attorney Jason. I related this situation, and he confirmed what was happening. Both Jason and I were told the hearing would be continued.

Paralegal Carol had asked for a continuance of our case. Attorney Kyle objected. The judge upheld this objection. Attorney Kyle had us in a checkmate position. There was nowhere to go.

The next day came. The final hearing was held. Attorney Kyle was present. However, no one was at the final hearing representing me. My procedural Attorney Andy was in Colorado. The case was over.

The Judge's Workers' Compensation Decision

We received the compensation order. It was not in our favor. The judge used the word prejudice against me, denied compensation, and so forth. It is obvious these terms did not bode well. The following is the compensation order from the judge:

> "The claimant's complaints and symptoms are more logically and more readily explained as a thyroid disease and psychiatric problems which clearly pre-existed (in the case of the psychiatric problems, at least) the formation of his professional association and his practice in Sarasota."

At this time, I was not aware that Attorney Kyle had used my medical history from Dr. Herman Birkner, my gastroenterologist, which stated that I took Librax in New Jersey for a stomach problem. They made the claim that I had a psychiatric problem because I stated to Dr. Birkner that I had once taken Librax.

It seems to me that it takes a wild stretch of imagination to clearly state that I had a psychiatric problem on the basis that I had once said to Dr. Birkner that I had taken Librax for a stomach problem! How did the judge arrive at this conclusion? What did the judge have against me for him not to make a clear assessment of my case?

As to the thyroid disease (hyperthyroidism), this was caused by my exposure to mercury. This has been well documented in the literature. The World Health Organization states that increased radioactive iodine uptake by the thyroid is one of the criteria in making a diagnosis of mercury toxicity. Trakhtenberg also did a study and found a significant increase of hyperthyroidism among mercury workers.

The following is a statement from Dr. Kuhnau, an immunologist at the American Biologics, dated August 17, 1987:

> "Dr. Stuart Scheckner was under my care at American Biologics Hospital in October of 1986.
>
> It is my medical opinion that his prior episode of hyperthyroidism was the result of mercury intoxication."

I believe this document was available during my case.

A rehearing was held the following week. I will never forget the following words from defense Attorney Kyle, which rang out in my ears:

> **"Dr. Scheckner probably had mercury poisoning for years. But the case is over. It's just too bad!"**

How could what happened be so clear to the attorney opposing me, yet the judge ruled against me?

My merits attorney, Jason, walked down the steps of the courthouse with me and my wife, and then to the corner of the block. He turned to us and said, "I am going to say something that I very rarely say. It is the big M-word, malpractice." He was referring to Attorney Andy, the attorney covering the legal procedural parts of my case. Attorney Andy was in Colorado at the time of the final hearing.

These were the other statements by the judge in the first final compensation order:

Page 6, paragraph 5: "Before 1978, the claimant by history, had episodes of anxiety and depression. He was treated medically for this and apparently suffered some intermittent period of disability." (Fact: Absolutely no disability prior to 1978, psychological or physical; must be referring to Librax.)

Page 6, paragraph 5: "In 1978 or 1979 he developed bad complaints of indigestion, insomnia, diarrhea, constipation, morbid depression, fearfulness, panic attacks, tachycardia, fatigue and palpitations or tremors in chest." (Fact: Mercury spill occurred in 1978. *The above symptoms are consistent with mercury toxicity.*)

I had a prominent lawyer, Attorney Francis Ebenger, review the above description of events. He said that since there was no one to represent me at the final hearing, the only evidence that the judge could use was that which was presented against me by Kyle, the attorney of the insurance company. So I did not have a chance in a difficult case.

Attorney Francis Ebenger's comment on Attorney Andy: "Gross malpractice!"

In addition, Attorney Ebenger makes the following comment: "Having served on the Cleveland, Ohio grievance committee for many years, I was appalled at the many legal malfunctions and mis-functions committed upon Dr. Scheckner."

Chapter 17

Second Workers' Compensation Case

Attorney Andy, who was covering the legal procedural part of my case, suggested that I file a new case. He asked whether I wanted to file on the basis of mercury toxicity and/or on a psychiatric basis. I told him that I wanted to file on the basis of mercury toxicity. I did not want to have a psychiatric label on me. I asked him if we could file a second time, and he answered in the affirmative.

After years of trying to put things together, I finally had what one would consider a strong case. I had Dr. Louis Chang, a world-renowned toxicologist, as my expert witness and a comprehensive report from Dr. Sandra Denton.

Attorney Kyle, the defense counsel for the workers' compensation insurance company, retained Dr. Bob* as an expert witness.

Dr. Bob gave a preliminary deposition on my case. Attorney Jason, who was covering the merits of my case, pointed out something in the deposition. Dr. Bob had indicated that if Dr. Scheckner had a spill of mercury in his carpet, the vacuum would have removed it, and then there would be no problem!

The following is a quote from Dr. Bob's deposition:

> "The depositions say that the office was cleaned 2 to 3 times a week with the vacuum. Based on that I would say that within a short period of time, within days, the majority of that mercury would have been sucked up and removed from the office.
>
> Carpeting tends to be a useful item to spill mercury onto, because it tends to contain it rather than to let it form a large surface area like any other physical phenomenon would be restricted, and it would make it much easier to clean it up."[15]

If we believe this type of unscientific reasoning which contradicts medical peer-reviewed literature, then Dr. Bob can make us believe anything he wants! There is a word for the quote above, "BS". How could the judge allow Dr. Bob to continue as an expert witness for the defense against me after this flagrant fabrication!?

The literature is very clear that shag carpeting is especially dangerous for mercury spills. "Contaminated carpeting . . . should be discarded after cleanup." In addition, the vacuum and the vacuum's housing, the motor, and all parts of the vacuum cleaner would be contaminated. Every time the vacuum runs, mercury would be dispersed. Changing the filter bag of the vacuum would not solve the problem. The vacuum would be a continual source of mercury contamination.[16]

Regarding Dr. Bob, he is not a toxicologist.

The following is a quote from Attorney Frank Recker:

> "Dr. Bob has largely made a career out of marketing himself as an 'expert witness' in both the medical and dental

---

[15] Deposition of Dr. Bob, DDS, MD, through telephone dated April 1, 1984, p. 19.

[16] U.S. Department of Health and Human Services, *Case Studies and Environmental Medicine, Mercury Toxicity* (March 1992), 16.

> professions, notwithstanding his relative lack of clinical experience in the actual practice of either profession."

Dr. Bob is a strong advocate of the safety of mercury-silver fillings: http://www.flcv.com/dams.html. Please see under "Medical Issues, Review . . ."

The following are quotes taken from Tim Bolen's site (http://www.quackpotwatch.org/):

> "Friday, January 26th, 2007 - Top 'quackbuster' Dr. Bob . . . MD, DDS PhD was forcibly removed as a witness in a California case recently after it was pointed out to the State of California that Dr. Bob was not quite what he claims to be. Cases all over the United States, originally initiated by 'quackbusters,' are being dropped by State agencies - like hot potatoes.
>
> For instance, Court Documents show:
>
> The sole purpose of the activities of B* & Dr. Bob . . . are to discredit and cause damage and harm to health care practitioners and businesses that make alternative health therapies or products available, and advocates of non-allopathic therapies and health freedom.
>
> Dr. Bob has various versions of his CV, with conflicting and inaccurate information.
>
> July 10th, 2003 - The Wisconsin trial (cross-examination) of Dr. Bob MD, DDS, PhD has been moved one day, and will now begin on July 15th, 2003, and extend through July 17th, 2003. Dr. Bob will be questioned, for three full days, on his credibility and the claims he made on his resume. Dr. Bob resume seems to be a fantasy world of his own devising, as investigation doesn't bear out his claims."

A telephone deposition was arranged for Rodman Shipman, MD. He is a psychiatrist. Dr. Roy Kupsinel had recommended him. I made an appointment to see Dr. Shipman. In a letter to me, he stated that I had mercury poisoning and did not need psychiatric therapy.

So we were at my attorney's office. We were ready for the telephonic deposition to take place. Dr. Shipman had allocated an hour of his valuable office time for us. My attorneys were present. We waited and waited. Attorney Kyle, the insurance attorney, never showed up! I believe that he purposely did not show up to avoid having a deposition that would be very favorable to me. Dr. Shipman was understandably annoyed that his time was wasted. Was this a game of chess, and I was the pawn being pushed around? Here was an important deposition that would have supported my case of mercury toxicity, and it was lost! Dr. Shipman would have made it very clear that I had mercury poisoning and not a psychiatric condition!

After consulting with several attorneys, I was informed that once the deposition above was scheduled at a time and place, my attorneys should have continued with the deposition irrespective of the defense attorney not showing up, especially since Dr. Shipman was a noted specialist setting aside time from his practice to be deposed. This is a flagrant example of clear incompetence as this deposition could have well meant me winning my workers' compensation case.

The defense attorneys were using very clever tactics to win the case. They employed Dr. Bob as their expert witness against me and eliminated Dr. Shipman, who was on my side. I thought to myself, *Can the same type of legal tactics be used to sentence a man to death*? Can the law process be so distorted that the truth and the fair legal practices become subverted?

We finally had a comprehensive medical report from Sandra Denton, MD. It was well documented with a great deal of medical information corroborating my claim that I had mercury toxicity. I had to fly across the United States from Sarasota, Florida, to Kent, Washington. I spent one week going through extensive testing. The summary statement was this: "This report is to attest to the fact that Stuart Scheckner, D.D.S., is indeed suffering from the results of mercury poisoning."

Chapter 18

Dr. Denton's Report

MEDICAL REPORT for Dr. STUART SCHECKNER (Abridged)

BY SANDRA DENTON, M. D, 4/30/90

"This report is to attest to the fact that Stuart Scheckner, D.D.S., is indeed suffering from the results of mercury poisoning.

Because of my expertise and knowledge in the area of mercury toxicity, Dr. Scheckner consulted me on September 26, 1988, in my office in Kent, Washington. *His symptoms were classic for mercury toxicity.* The most distressing symptom was "internal tremors" which he describes as facial muscles taut and chest and body in constant tremor. He felt horrible and was in agony minute by minute from this particular symptom. He also had tremor of the extremities which was evident on his handwriting and when holding a piece of paper. Other symptoms included frequent urination (several times during the night), chronic cough (which produced a metallic taste), respirations which were uncomfortable and strained, extreme irritability, constipation accompanied by anal fissures and hemorrhoids (previously had diarrhea), nausea, difficulty thinking and concentrating, numbness dorsum right wrist, areas of burning on skin which when rubbed turn bright red (dermatographia), dizziness upon changing position from sitting to standing, weight loss in past (165 to 125), indecision, blurring vision, cramping of feet, slight buzzing of ears, unexplained anxiety spells where "he felt like he was going to die in the next minute" and "like climbing the walls (this symptom was only 5-10% of what it used to be), migratory joint pains, hands swollen right worse than left, digestive disorder after each meal even when drinking water, tachycardia, exhaustion (better now than used to be), burning sensation of mouth, difficulty sleeping because of the tremor sensation, cold hands and feet. Physical exam: B.P. 106/72 supine 118/82 stranding T. 98 P 68 R16 5'8" 151 lbs. Cold hands/feet; decreased hair distribution lower extremities, decreased lateral- 1/3 of eyebrows, coated tongue with scalloped edges, composite fillings, tremor of hands, heart/ lungs ok, abdominal muscles slight tremor to palpation, neck normal size. Additional tests recommended were:

1) adrenal stimulation test – "adrenal exhaustion" with marked deficiency of dehydroepiandrosterone pre and post ACTH stimulation and abnormal post stimulation result for tetrahydrocortisone. The abnormal- DHEA result night explain the severe muscle weakness. It is a well known fact that mercury accumulates in the adrenal glands and causes cellular dysfunction. This is an additional target organ which has been damaged by mercury poisoning.
2) fasting serum amino acid profile- deficiency of several essential amino acids, particularly sulfur containing amino acids taurine, threonine, glutamine which are often associated with tremors. It is documented that mercury binds with sulfur amino acids creating deficiencies. Taurine deficiency has also been associated with cardiac dysrhythmias and seizure disorders as it is known to regulate the electrical activity of the heart and brain.
3) serum compatibility test for dental materials - demonstrated an adverse immune response to mercury, copper, and aluminum.
4) Thyroid microsomal antibody – abnormal elevation → autoimmune thryroiditis.

I have spent approximately 30 hours reviewing Dr. Scheckner's medical records. The following portion of the report contains what I feel are the pertinent facts in this case.

Not only was Dr. Scheckner occupationally exposed from the practice of dentistry beginning in 1964 and continuing until his forced medical retirement in April, 1984, but he was additionally exposed when a full bottle of mercury was accidentally spilled onto the shag carpet in his operatory in 1978 by his assistant, Linda. The entire contents of the bottle were lost in the carpeting. None of the mercury could be retrieved. Since Linda had no formal training, she did not realize the seriousness of the incident, nor did she have any idea of the hazard which she created for those who worked in that room.

The mercury spill occurred at the base of the dental chair, where the assistant stood, and her feet agitated the spilled mercury in the carpet, causing an increased vaporization. Furthermore the carpet was vacuumed twice a week, further agitating the mercury in the shag and enhancing vaporization.

"The silent hazard: An unusual case of mercury contamination of a dental suite" by Leonard Pagnotto, Vol. 92, June '76, p. 1195, describes a mercury spill in a dental office, caused by vandals. Unaware of the possibility of agitation of the mercury vapor in the rug, the dental assistants had regularly vacuumed the rugs. By doing so they unsuspectingly subjected themselves to mercury vapor escaping through the fabric of the collector bag of the vacuum, as well as to the mercury that was recirculated in the air by the vacuuming.

Replacement of the rugs did not solve the situation, because the old vacuum cleaner was still being used. Even though a new bag had been obtained, using a mercury-vapor meter it was found that the motor housing was heavily contaminated with mercury. Heat from the motor, of course, readily vaporized the mercury, and the people in the office became ill until the cause was found, and removed.

The case of Stuart Scheckner directly parallels the JADA report. Furthermore, in the summer the air conditioning in Dr. Scheckner's office was turned off on weekends, allowing temperatures to exceed

95 degrees Fahrenheit, again enhancing the vaporization of the spilled mercury. The heavily contaminated area existed in his office for at least one year, until the rug was removed as a suspected cause of the prevailing illness in office personnel. One hygienist, in fact, had to seek medical attention because of symptoms of tachycardia, constipation alternating with diarrhea, nausea, headache, and abdominal pains.

The following years were evidently pure hell for Dr. Scheckner. He continued losing weight; in 1982 he developed tachycardia and consulted Dr. Gene Meyers (cardiologist), who performed a stress EKG and interpreted everything as normal, and prescribed valium which had no effect on the tachycardia (fast heart beat). During a hernia operation in 1982 the tachycardia was again documented, and an elevated T4 was found. Dr. Scheckner consulted Dr. Hope-Gill, who diagnosed his condition as "Graves' Disease." He was placed on medication (Ativan and Inderal) but continued to suffer, even though the T4 returned to normal.

Since then Wolfram Kuhnau, M.D. has attested that the "Graves' Disease" was most likely mercury's effect on the thyroid gland. Dr. Scheckner's thyroid I123 uptake was abnormally increased, measuring 58.6% at 24 hours, on 9/2/82. In September 1988 Dr. Scheckner had abnormal thyroid antibodies. (Thyroid microsomal antibodies 400; normal is 0-99, confirming an autoimmune thyroiditis.)

Several reports have indicated that both the pituitary and thyroid glands display an affinity for accumulating mercury in humans. (Suzuki et al. 1966 Affinity of Hg to the thyroid. INDUSTRIAL HEALTH 4, 69-75) Concentration of mercury in thyroid and pituitary glands were much higher than that observed in kidney, brain, or liver tissue in people working in mercury mines in Slovenia, Yugoslavia. *(Kosta et al. 1975 Correlation between selenium and Hg in men following exposure to inorganic Hg. NATURE LONDON 254, 238-239)*

The British medical journal LANCET reports the extremely high concentrations of mercury in the pituitary glands of dentists compared with control populations.

Another article speaks on the interference on the synthesis of T3 exerted by mercury. This backup could explain an elevated T4. This article states that these changes may be permanent and irreversible, and appear to be related to the quantity of mercury administered, and the length of time during which the exposure to mercury persists. (The effect of HgCl on thyroid function in the rat. Goldman & Blackburn, TOXICOLOGY & APPLIED PHARMACOLOGY 48, 49-55 1979)

There are numerous references in the literature linking mercury as a causative agent in autoimmune diseases.

In Casarett & Doull's TOXICOLOGY, THE BASIC SCIENCE OF POISONING, p. 608, with chronic exposure to mercury vapor, the major effects are on the central nervous system. Early signs are non-specific and have been termed the "asthenic vegetative syndrome" or "micromercurialism." Identification of the syndrome requires neurasthenic symptoms and 3 or more of the following clinical findings:

- * Tremor
- Enlargement of the thyroid
- * Increased uptake of radioiodine in the thyroid
- * Labile pulse
- * Tachycardia
- * Dermographism
- * Gingivitis
- * Hematologic changes
- Increased excretion of mercury in the urine

*(Dr. Scheckner fulfills 7 requirements, preceded by [*], above.)*

In September 1987, Dr. Scheckner had an electroencephalogram by Ron, M.D. which was abnormal. The report stated, "intermittent periods of paroxysmal high amplitude bursts of theta activity in the 5 to 7 Hz range, which emanated out of normal background and were generalized. On one occasion the patient felt "internal vibrations." These results are similar to those reported in the article, "Late EEG Findings and Clinical Status After Organic Hg poisoning." (Richard

Brenner, M.D. & Russell Snyder, M.D. ARCH NEUROL VOL 37 May 1980 282-284.) According to the article, "the degree of EEG change reflected the clinical state. Various types of abnormalities were noted, including epileptiform features and disturbances of background rhythms. Bursts of theta activity were present diffusely. Diffuse slowing of background rhythm usually of 6 to 7 Hertz, which was reactive to eye-opening and eye-closing. Abnormalities were present nearly 10 years after poisoning."

Dr. Scheckner had a quantitative Topographic EEG by Dr. James A. Lewis, Sarasota Palms, Florida, on 3/16/89, which was also abnormal and was consistent with "mild to moderate encephalopathy." It is my medical opinion that these two abnormal EEG's are adequate objective documentation of mercury poisoning on Stuart Scheckner's central nervous system.

Dr. Scheckner was required to have a psychological evaluation was part of his disability determination. This was done by Rona W. Ross, Ph.D., in Sarasota, Florida in December 1985. Tests done at that time included Canter BIP Bender, WAIS-R, Memory tasks, Figure Drawing, and Rorschach. Results showed tremors at rest and when writing, and in all of his reproduction, organic brain damage, erratic memory function, impairment of intellectual functioning, perceptual motor deficiency, leading to diagnosis of *"possible dementia related to mercury toxicity."* Dr. Ross reports "no psychogenic basis" for Dr. Scheckner's problems. In other words, Dr. Scheckner's problem was not "all in his head."

This is consistent with the findings of Dr. Joel Butler, Ph. D., Professor of Psychology, University of North Texas. Dr. Butler has 26 years of teaching experience and research, and is the author of over 100 publications including co-authorship in 10 books on psychology. Dr. Butler has spent several years studying perceptual motor skills and the psychological profile of dentists in general. A battery of tests in this area brings the effects of mercury on dental personnel into focus. His preliminary test results show that neuro-psychological dysfunction was present in 90% of the dentists tested.

Dr. Butler's work appears in the *Proceedings of the International Conference of Biocompatibility of Materials*, published by Life Science Press in Tacoma, WA in 1989.

On two occasions, Dr. Scheckner had excessive amounts of mercury on tissue analysis of hair samples (11/20/84 -- 15 ppm, 6/20/85 – 18.2 ppm.) According to Goldwater in 1964, hair mercury levels in the general population averages 1.2 to 4.2 ppm. An expert committee from Sweden established an upper limit of 6 ppm for hair mercury.

This was during a time that Dr. Scheckner was receiving intravenous chelation treatments. EDTA chelation mobilizes Hg from the blood and assists in excretion of mercury and other heavy metals. During chelation treatments Dr. Scheckner's symptoms improved but returned after the IV's were discontinued. This was a diagnostic tool further strengthening the diagnosis of "Heavy Metal Toxicity," noticeably mercury.

Since these results were after Dr. Scheckner had ceased working his dental practice, the elevated figures cannot be attributed to external contamination.

Dr. Scheckner's tachycardia and heart disturbances have evidently been continuous, from earliest reports up to the present. An echocardiogram was done in 4/86, and was read as normal. There are many studies showing the accumulation of mercury in the heart causing an irregular heart rate.

In reviewing the many laboratory tests that Dr. Scheckner had over the years, I saw a predominance of abnormal results which include elevated eosinophils, intermittently elevated liver enzymes, elevated hemoglobin, and hematocrit values, fluctuations of glucose levels and abnormally low cholesterol levels. Each of these abnormalities has been associated with heavy metal toxicity, more specifically mercury.

His case has been contested because of the absence of elevated urine mercury levels. Most physicians would like to be able to diagnose mercury toxicity by finding a high urinary level of mercury. This idea has been found to be incorrect due to misinformation of the physiology of mercury in the body. High urine levels may be found in acute exposures (macromercurialsim). However, they are rarely present in the chronic low-dose exposures (micromercurialism). The chapter on mercury in the fifth edition of Clinical Toxicology of Commercial Products by Robert Gosselin, M.D., Ph.D.; and Harold Hodge, Ph.D., D.Sc., makes this clear. "Urinary mercury levels are characteristically low in chronic exposure suggesting a hypersensitivity reaction."

Another article by L. J. Goldwater, "The Toxicology of Inorganic Mercury" (Annals N.Y. Acad. Sci 65:498-503, 1957) says that urinary mercury levels may give some indication of the degree of exposure. However, they are of limited value in the diagnosis of poisoning. High levels can be found in human subjects who are symptoms free, and low levels in those exhibiting marked evidence of micromercurialism. It has been suggested that, in some cases, failure to excrete mercury is a factor in the development of poisoning.

T.W. Clarkson in Biological Monitoring of Toxic Metals, discusses the significance of urine mercury values: "Urinary excretion of mercury is used widely in monitoring workers exposed to mercury vapor (see U.S. EPA, 1984). However, the relationship between urinary excretion and absorbed dose is not well understood; urinary excretion may be directly related to the kidney burden of mercury unless renal damage has occurred." This point was also made by Lamm and Pratt in their 1985 study ("Subclinical Effects of Exposure to Inorganic Mercury Revealed by Somatosensory-Evoked Potentials" Eur Neurol 24:237-243, 1985) when they discovered a clear, negative and significant correlation between time on the job and the level of mercury in the urine. These researchers found that the longer a worker was on the job, the less mercury is excreted in his urine.

Poisoning by Arena and Drew, Fifth Edition, 1986, Toxicology - Symptoms – Treatment points out on p. 202-203 the error in relying on urine mercury for determination of toxicity. "The amount of mercury excreted in the urine, however, seemingly bears no direct relationship to the severity of symptoms. One must conclude that the response to mercurial exposure is to a great extent based, as it is with drugs in general, on individual sensitivity. The mercury level in the blood is a less reliable indicator of the degree of exposure than the mercury level of the urine. There is a rapid loss of mercury from the bloodstream after absorption and a variation in mercury levels of the urine. In individual cases, symptoms of poisoning is poor. Some with signs of poisoning may have lower mercury levels in the urine or blood than those without signs of poisoning. The diagnosis of mercury poisoning must be based on the history of exposure and physical examination, with secondary reliance on mercury level in the urine or blood, or both."

Blood levels are NOT helpful in the diagnosis of mercury poisoning because mercury remains in the blood for only a few minutes, after exposure. Mercury quickly finds its way into the various tissues of the body, depositing in the brain, adrenals, thyroid, and other organ systems. Only at high levels of exposure will this blood – level parameter be of any value.

We are indeed grateful to the work of Dr. Alfred Stock in the 1920's who reported much on his finding concerning mercury toxicity. He states that when air containing small amounts of mercury is inhaled, it will take a long time until the poisoning becomes apparent. From one to several years, these symptoms can be restricted to tiredness and slow deterioration of the intellectual ability and memory. In some cases reported in the literature, the symptoms reached their peak a few months after the patients were no longer exposed to mercury. Also, it is important to note that the recovery from insidious mercury poisoning after elimination of the poisonous source is extremely slow and there are often relapses. This is quite typical and has certainly been seen in the case of Dr. Scheckner.

Combined with previous tests and clinical histories, there should be little doubt that Dr. Scheckner is suffering from mercury poisoning. I agree with Nicholas Alexiou, M.D., Occupational Medicine, University of South Florida, College of Medicine who in March 1988 said there appears to be no explanation other than mercury poisoning to account for Dr. Scheckner's multiple symptoms. Furthermore, it would be unlikely that he can ever hope to return to the dental office to perform his skilled trade as a dentist. Mercury is ubiquitous in the dental office and the slightest exposure causes immediate exacerbation of all of his symptoms.

Because Dr. Scheckner's exposure continued so long before it was recognized and because of physicians' unfamiliarity with the condition of mercury poisoning, it is most likely that his neurological symptoms may be irreversible. At this time, Dr. Stuart Scheckner is unable to perform the required tasks demanded of any profession or occupation, and in my professional opinion I do not believe that rehabilitation in any vocation is possible.

Re: ENCYCLOPEDIA OF OCCUPATIONAL HEALTH & SAFETY, International Labour Office, Geneva, Vol. 2, 3rd edition, p. 1333: "If excessive exposure is not corrected, neuro-vegetative manifestations (tremor, sweating, dermatographia) become more pronounced associated with characterial and personality disorders and perhaps digestive disorders, (stomatitis, diarrhea) and a deterioration in general status anorexia, weight loss). Once this stage has been reached termination of exposure may not lead to full recovery."

It is indeed tragic that Dr. Stuart Scheckner's life and career have been so devastated by his occupational exposure to mercury. It is hoped that much can be learned from his unfortunate experience to prevent similar catastrophe from occurring in other dental personnel.

It is my medical opinion, within reasonable medical certainty, that the statements I have made regarding etiology (causation), condition and prognosis of Dr. Stuart Scheckner are as stated in this report."

Chapter 19

Matter of Medical Opinion or Fact?

I met a judge from Canada, and we were comparing our legal systems. I told him about my workers' compensation case and the ordeal I had gone through. He stated, "You have an adversarial system. In Canada, you would have had just consideration."

Since no urine mercury levels had been performed at the time of the spill, I was left in a very difficult situation in order to prove mercury toxicity in my workers' compensation case.

The only indication of mercury in my body was high mercury levels in my hair. This was determined by two separate independent laboratories. On November 20, 1984, Mineral Lab Inc. performed a hair element analysis on me. The result was a mercury level of 18 parts per million. Under the remarks section of the report was listed the notation of this level as "HIGHLY TOXIC." Stamped on the laboratory results paper was the statement "CONFIRMED BY REPEAT ANALYSIS."

On June 20, 1985, Parmae Laboratories performed a hair analysis test on a new hair sample. The results were shown on a color-shaded graph. The mercury level exceeded the limit in the graph. The reading given was 1.82. On the paper was stated, "ALL RESULTS IN mg/100gm (mg%)." In order to convert milligrams percent into parts per million, you multiply the figure by 10. This makes the amount 18.2 parts per million. Attached to this paper is the following statement:

> MERCURY
> HAIR LEVELS ARE HIGH. ELEVATED LEVELS OF MERCURY IN THE HAIR HAVE BEEN ASSOCIATED WITH HUMAN TOXICITY (PHELPS ET AL, 1980).

A horizontal line went through the 8 in 1.82 mg/% and made the 8 difficult to read. I asked Parmae Lab to write a statement on the mercury concentration in my hair. Parmae Lab sent me a letter stating my mercury value. This paper confirmed the reading of 1.82 mg%. It stated that you could convert the figure into parts per million by multiplying it by 10. Hence, 1.82 mg% x 10 = 18.2 parts per million.

The facts, therefore, indicate that two different independent laboratories performed hair analysis on samples taken a few months apart. As can be seen from the results, both labs reported high toxic mercury levels in my hair.

Since no urine mercury level was taken by any of my physicians during the exposure period, I was left in a very precarious position. If the attorneys of the insurance company could just negate my only evidence of personal exposure, my claim for compensation from mercury toxicity would be severely hurt.

Dr. Chang had recommended that I see Dr. Mal* before the insurance company's attorneys contacted him. Dr. Mal was a prestigious professor of neurology at a prominent medical school. He has since passed away. I had not attached a note of urgency to Dr. Chang's recommendation.

Then I was notified by Attorney Kyle that they had arranged for me to be examined by Dr. Mal. It was too late for me to get to Dr. Mal first. He had been retained by Attorney Kyle, not by me. I had no idea what I was in for. Was I going to get a fair shake or not?

I was early for my appointment with Dr. Mal. Immediately upon meeting him, I became aware that I was in an adversarial situation.

There was nothing I could do or say that would convince this man of my problem. He was retained by the insurance company's attorneys. As he performed his tests on me and questioned me, he chortled to himself. I will never forget Dr. Mal's mocking attitude toward me. The situation was like a cat and mouse game, and I was the mouse!

After the exam, I walked to the corridor. I stood there for about a minute or two. I then walked back to the examination room. The door was locked. I was looking for Dr. Mal, but he was nowhere to be found. I wanted to confront him and say, "What just happened here? Are you going to give me a fair shake, or are you going to make me look like a fool?" Then again, that might just have irritated him.

Dr. Mal wrote a letter to Dr. Ron, my neurologist, regarding my case:

> "The patient had hair samples measured on 11/24/84 by the Mineral Lab Incorporated in Hayward, California and it was felt that the mercury in his hair was 15 with a normal being less than 2.5. Subsequently from the ***same*** laboratory the hair was measured at 1.82 parts per million."

The above statement disagrees with the statements from the labs.

Dr. Mal stated that there was only one lab involved. The fact was that there were two! He stated that my hair mercury level in that *one* lab was 15 parts per million and, subsequently, 1.82 parts per million, normal being less than 2.5. He was stating, therefore, that the 1.82 value was less than the 2.5 value, making it normal and not toxic. These facts were so critical to my case in proving my exposure. *Dr. Mal misquoted the value by saying it was 1.82 parts per million. It was 1.82 mg/%, which is a toxic level of 18.2 parts per million.* In the Parmae Lab report, on the fourth column from the right, was the graphic level of mercury. You could see the vertical extension of the asterisks, which denoted the level of toxicity. The vertical asterisks maxed out the column. How could this level even be considered low even if one mistook the relationship of mg/% (milligrams percent) with ppm (parts per million)?

The following are the reports from the *two* laboratories. Both labs showed high mercury levels. How could a brilliant professor make such a bad mistake as to say a second lab test showed hair mercury level was normal and that the first one was a mistake? This flies in the face of the facts:

Mercury in Hair

11/20/84	Mineral Lab	15 parts per million
6/20/85	Parmae Lab	1.82 mg/% = 18.2 parts per million

Dr. Mal has written peer-reviewed documents. He is a prestigious author on various neurological subjects, including mercury toxicity. He has written on the effects of mercury vapor intoxication. His paper states the following: "The defects in memory suggest involvement of the *temporal lobes*."[17]

Dr. Ron, a neurologist, documented *temporal lobe* dysfunction in me. The first medical report diagnosing temporal lobe involvement was from him, who, I believe, was a student of Dr. Mal at the medical school. Dr. Ron's statement was this: "Impressions: abnormal electroencephalogram, classification III (highly significant), on the basis of the notation of intermittent slowing and disorganization in the bi-*temporal* regions, with associated frequent single spike-like discharges. This recording is consistent with cortical irritability *bi-temporally*, with associated encephalopathy."

This above medical report by Dr. Ron was sent to Dr. Mal for his review.

It is amazing that in the "Mercury Vapor Intoxication" report prepared by Dr. Mal, temporal lobe involvement was mentioned ten times![18] Therefore, my documented temporal lobe dysfunction by Dr. Ron was not a frivolous finding. Although Dr. Mal *did not* diagnose temporal lobe dysfunction in me, his former student *did*!

---

[17] Citation truncated to hide identity,Brain (1972),Mercury Vapour Intoxication, p. 315.

[18] Citation truncated to hide identity, Brain (1972),Mercury Vapour Intoxication, p. 308, 309, 311, 315, 316, 317.

The following is a letter that I received from Parmae Lab clarifying the results:

> "Parmae Laboratories
> August 27, 1990
>
> TO WHOM IT MAY CONCERN:
>
> This is to verify that on June 20, 1985 Parmae Laboratories ran a hair analysis on Stuart Scheckner, DDS. The resulting analysis revealed an extremely high Mercury reading of 1.82 milligrams percent (mgs %). Milligrams percent refers to milligrams per 100 grams of hair. If you wish to convert milligrams percent to parts per million (ppm), you multiply by ten.
>
> Sincerely,
> Agnes Horvat, Ph.D.
> Laboratory Director"

A letter was sent from Dr. Mal to Dr. Ron. Subsequent to this letter, Dr. Ron gave a deposition on my case. The room was small and dimly lit and had a rectangular table. A number of people were sitting around the table. My Attorney Jason asked a question regarding mercury. Dr. Ron quickly dismissed the issue, and it was never brought up again. The deposition seemed to be lengthy. I was hoping to hear Dr. Ron state that I had temporal lobe dysfunction, which could be related to mercury toxicity. I expected this since he had given me this information on my first appointment; however, he never brought up this critical information. My feeling is that Dr. Mal negatively influenced his former student Dr. Ron against me to not relate mercury and his own finding of temporal lobe dysfunction.

Several years after this report by Dr. Mal, a new EEG was performed by Dr. George Rozelle on July 17, 1996. It stated, "Impression: This EEG supports earlier findings of temporal lobe abnormalities."

I had a total of six brain function tests using an EEG over a number of years. There were five reports of abnormal brain function. *The only normal interpretation was that of Dr. Mal.* He was retained by the attorneys of the insurance company. How can a renowned professor of neurology distort the facts given above? I am sadly disillusioned about the ethics of a renowned doctor of medicine. It seems money can be above ethics. Perhaps, I have been too naïve. How can this distortion of truth be possible in the medical profession!?

Dr. Mal's medical opinion was in contradiction to Dr. Louis Chang's, a world-renowned toxicologist, and Dr. Sandra Denton's, who did an extensive medical work-up on me.

The following is one of the abnormal brain function reports:

Centre for Neurological Evaluation
ELECTROENCEPALOGRAPHY
DONALD NEGROSKI, M.D.

Name: STUART SCHECKNER Age: 52
Referring Physician: Negroski
EEG Number: 90-270 Date: 12/20/90

Clinical History: Mercury toxicity

CLASSIFICATION: Abnormal, Significance I (mildly significant).

1. Intermittent slow, generalized rare.
2. Prolonged intermittent theta, after hyperventilation was discontinued.

INTERPRETATION:

This 3-minute awake and Stage II sleep electroencephalogram demonstrates slowing as noted above, suggesting a mild diffuse encephalopathy. The etiology of this is non-specific, but may be seen in degenerative, toxic, metabolic, or primary degenerative disorders. Clinical correlation is needed. Epileptiform activity was not identified on this tracing.

Donald Negroski, M.D.

cc: Dr. Scheckner

Chapter 20

The Final Hearing

I picked up Dr. Chang from the Sarasota airport. One of the first things that we did was go to the hospital to obtain my last EEG for temporal lobe dysfunction. When Dr. Chang read the results of the test, he stated it was like a fingerprint of mercury poisoning!

From a standpoint of credentials, I was in a very good position. I had one of the leading world toxicologists, Louis Chang, PhD, as my expert witness. Dr. Chang explained to me that my EEG conformed to the picture of mercury toxicity. Furthermore, I fulfilled the criteria of the World Health Organization:

> "Studies related assessment of the occurrence of so-called asthenic vegetative syndrome or "micromercurialism" have been reported by I.M. Trakhtenberg. This syndrome may occur in persons with or without mercury exposure. For a diagnosis of mercury induced asthenic vegetative syndrome, I.M. Trakhtenberg reviewed by Friberg & Nordberg, 1972, required that not only neurasthenic symptoms should be present but as supporting evidence three or more of the following clinical findings: *tremor*, enlargement of the thyroid, *increased uptake of radio-iodine in the thyroid, labile pulse, tachycardia, dermatographism,*

> *gingivitis, haemotological* changes, and excretion of mercury in the urine which was above normal or increased 8-fold after medication with unithiol."[19]

I must have been brainwashed by the ADA. I had performed an IV DMPS urine mercury challenge test. The pre-challenge result was undetectable (detection limit 2). The post-challenge result was 11 ugHg/liter (micrograms of mercury per liter). In prior urine mercury levels, the results were close to 0. Therefore, there could have been a much greater increase than the eight-fold requirement of supporting evidence. However, I was looking for 150 ugHg/liter, which the ADA stated was necessary to show toxicity. This information never got to Dr. Chang, who might have been able to use it for me. I was not altogether thinking too clearly with my condition.

It was the date of the hearing. Dr. Chang and Dr. Denton were there to testify on my behalf. I believed that Dr. Denton's comprehensive report and analysis of my condition were critical in supporting my condition. Her conclusion was I had a classic case of mercury poisoning. Dr. Chang would provide the scientific expertise to support these findings. I remember standing in the corridor outside the hearing room with Dr. Chang and Dr. Denton at my sides. I felt that I finally had the support I needed to validate what had happened to me. Dr. Bob was there representing the insurance company.

The defense attorneys had found Linda, my former secretary who had spilled mercury in my shag carpeting in 1978. She denied spilling the mercury. The incident happened 12 years ago, and she did not have any recollection of it. As I explained earlier, I never made an issue of this incident with her at the time, and I therefore believe that this occurrence was of little consequence to her. She was not a trained assistant and was therefore totally unaware of the danger posed by a large spill of mercury.

---

19 Environmental Health Criteria 1, Mercury, Published under the joint sponsorship of the United Nations Environment Programme and the World Health Organization (Geneva, 1976): 91.

The defense attorney was effectively dismissing my exposure to mercury both with the testimony of Linda and with the statement from Dr. Mal that I did not have high levels of mercury in my hair. This, of course, went against the facts in front of him. If Dr. Mal had openly stated the fact that my hair mercury levels were high, it would have given me a much better chance of a just outcome of my case. I remember that Dr. Chang had told me to see Dr. Mal before the insurance company's attorney had contacted him. Perhaps if I had taken Dr. Chang's advice, Dr. Mal's opinion would have been supportive and impartial.

I went into the hearing room for a few minutes. I vaguely remember the judge being sarcastic to Dr. Denton, implying that she was one of those way-out alternative medical physicians. I was quite nervous at this point and went outside the hearing room in the corridor and waited.

After quite some time, I was called into the hearing room. The judge asked me what my problem was. I stupidly answered that I had constipation. I was so nervous, and I froze and did not know how to respond. How would I express verbally what I was going through and have the judge really understand it? I had about thirty-five symptoms, the worst being morbid agitation with internal tremors, that of climbing the walls, a most horrible feeling, but he did not hear that. The judge had all the documents with all my symptoms and medical reports. During the time that I was in the hearing room, my credibility was attacked. They were really trying to get me from all angles.

All the years of going through an adversarial legal process were now over. The judge made his ruling. He not only denied me compensation but also allowed the insurance carrier's attorney to file for taxation of costs. In other words, the judge allowed Attorney Kyle to be compensated for their expenses. He ordered me to pay $13,846.74 to the employer or the carrier. Attorney Roz*, an associate of attorney Andy, wrote, "Neither Andy nor I have seen costs awarded in a workers' compensation case during all the time we have been practicing." Attorney Jason protested and filed to have the insurance carrier's attorney document the expenses. Rather than go through the trouble, they agreed to accept $5,000 only if paid within the day. Otherwise, I was told they would just about go for everything that I had. I gave them a check for $5,000 the next day. What an ordeal and a nightmare with my workers' compensation, and I was still suffering from mercury toxicity!

With regard to the merits of the case, the judge stated that I had a psychiatric disorder prior to my incorporation in the State of Florida. He based this on a medical record from Dr. Herman Birkner, a gastroenterologist to whom I had stated that I had taken Librax for a stomach problem one time. In a letter that I later requested from Dr. Hurewitz, my New Jersey family physician, this allegation was refuted. Subsequent to the loss of my case, I wrote a letter to Dr. Hurewitz. Dr. Hurewitz sent me a letter stating, "My memory is quite clear regarding Stuart's emotional state. He had always been a well adjusted healthy young man with a bright future." In addition, Dr. Hurewitz stated, "I do not recall prescribing Librax, a medication which is usually used by gastroenterologists even now in the treatment of peptic ulcers. I have *never* seen or heard of it being prescribed for emotional states or adjustment disorders. If I did prescribe it, it must have been for a mild upper Gastrointestinal irritation, the symptomatic short-term treatment."

The judge also stated that my problem was due to a thyroid disorder. Dr. Chang had surely covered this. Prior to the hearing, Dr. Chang had recommended that I see an endocrinologist to rule out Graves' disease. Dr. Antunes, an endocrinologist, ran tests on me to confirm that my thyroid was normal. Here again was another distortion of the facts. The judge stated that I had thyroid disease even though it had been ruled out.

I remember very clearly Dr. Chang's remark after I lost my case. He said, "The judge played doctor!" I do not believe that Dr. Chang had ever lost a case as an expert witness before mine. I believe that he, one of the most respected and world-renowned toxicologists, took on my case because he respected me for standing up for my rights and believed that there was no question that I had occupational mercury toxicity.

The only bright spot of this whole workers' compensation case was that I met Dr. Louis Chang. After the loss of my case, I visited Dr. Chang in Little Rock, Arkansas. He is an amazing man. He is very witty and intelligent. I am honored that he considers me his friend.

During my case, I was in communication with Florida Governor Lawton Chiles. He seemed to be following my case closely. I have the highest respect and regard for Governor Chiles. He seemed a very kind and sympathetic man. I think he was a great governor of the State of Florida. In the last letter I received from him, he stated that if it's any "consolation for you," I did not reappoint the judge as a hearing officer for Sarasota. I have always thought well of Governor Chiles, and his caring consideration for me was very much appreciated.

A few months after the loss of my workers' compensation case, I met my merits attorney, Jason, at an Office Depot. He said that he had spoken to the judge about my case. Jason said that the judge admitted that he probably had made a mistake in my case. I asked what could be done. Jason said, "Nothing!"

Sometime after the loss of my workers' compensation case, I met Susan, my former dental assistant, at the gym where I had worked out. I told her about the case.

The following is a statement from Susan many years later, too late to make a difference, which appeared in a local newspaper:

> "I was given explicit instructions to be careful in handling the dental mercury. I was told about the large spill of mercury that occurred before my employment . . . I was concerned about exposure. I brought in a mercury detector badge and placed it in the office. The badge turned dark gray at an extremely fast rate, indicating a high level of mercury vapor."

This photo of the mercury detector did not surface till many years later. Susan could have testified. She said, "Don't you remember the mercury detector that I placed in your operatory?" Evidently, I did not.

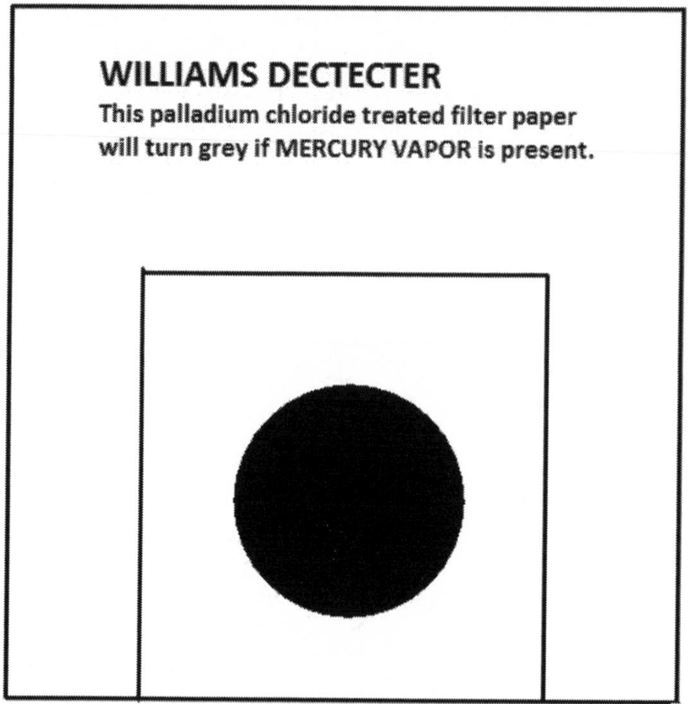

The mercury vapor present in Dr. Scheckner's office changed this detector to nearly black.

This evidence could have proven my exposure to mercury, but it did not enter my mind through the years of my ordeal with the workers' compensation case. Professor Stock said it succinctly: "Quem Mercurius perdere vult, dementat prius!" (Whom Mercury wants to destroy, he first robs of his mind!)

To Rub Salt into a Wound

After the case was finished, it was clear that malpractice had been committed. I consulted an attorney who took the malpractice case on. He notified attorney Andy who had committed the malpractice that I intended to sue him. That attorney told him that unless I gave him $500 that he would begin to sue me for improper pleadings and cost me a lot of time and money. My attorney who I had hired advised me to give him the $500 to avoid this litigation which on his advice I did. When I told this to attorney Francis Ebenger, he could not believe it. After all the legal malpractice and injustices committed on me to this time, this was the worst of all. Attorney Ebenger can see how people can have a bad taste in their mouth regarding the legal system and attorneys from Dr. Scheckner's horrid experience.

Chapter 21

History of Dental Amalgam

Since the American Dental Association was wrong about me, is it possible that they are also wrong about the danger of mercury in the common mercury-silver filling, the fillings you may have in your mouth?

How did we first start using mercury as a filling material in dentistry? I will use the term *dental amalgam* and *mercury-silver fillings* interchangeably as they are the same.

In the 1800's, gold became popular as a dental filling material. Beaten gold leaf was used to fill a dental cavity. Its use was limited since there had to be four strong walls for the gold leaf to be compressed against. Non-cohesive gold needed four strong walls of the tooth so that enough pressure could be applied so it would hold together.

Then, in 1855, Dr. Robert A. Arthur discovered the cohesiveness of gold foil. "Arthur found that cohesion could be induced by the simple process of passing the gold foil over a spirit flame, after which it could be welded cold."[20] While I was in dental school, we were taught the

[20] M. D. K. Bremner, *The Story of Dentistry* (Brooklyn, New York, 1958), 242.

gold foil technique. My brother has a sample of my work while I was a dental student. It is a difficult and time-consuming procedure, which is very rarely performed today, if at all. "It was a fine operation when well done, but nerve wracking for the dentist and brutal for the patient. Very few will mourn its passing into oblivion."[21] During the 1800's, gold was very expensive, and the technique was quite difficult. Many people just could not afford this filling.

Many different materials were tried, but most of them had too many problems. Silver was too stiff and was not ductile enough to be compressed into the cavity. It was not malleable like gold. Tin, platinum, and aluminum were some of the other materials experimented on but did not work out.

Fusible metals were used, such as an alloy of tin, lead, and bismuth. A small amount of mercury was added to hasten the fusing to lower the melting point to 212 degrees Fahrenheit. This alloy was melted and then poured into the cavity. I wonder how the patient endured a hot molten metal in their open cavity.

Later, more mercury was added to this fusible alloy. This lowered the melting point to 140 degrees. The technique differed in that small pieces of the alloy would be placed in the cavity. The pieces of alloy would be fused together with a hot instrument.

The time was ripe for someone who had an answer to filling teeth that most people could afford.

The "Crawcour incident": In 1833, the Crawcour brothers came to the United States with a cheap coin silver amalgam. This was a mixture of mercury and a silver powder. They called it "royal mineral succedaneum." This term was a substitute for the royal mineral gold. They had learned a "superficial knowledge" of dentistry in France. They were entrepreneurs who wanted to capitalize on this new filling material in the United States. They set up practice in New York and

---

21 Ibid., 243.

made a lot of money. Their "poor dentistry" and competition with other dentists created a lot of publicity.

Many other dentists started using amalgam since it was easy to use and cheap. As more dentists used amalgam, other dentists used it as well to meet the competition. Therefore, the use of dental amalgam quickly spread.

In 1841, the American Society of Dental Surgeons was formed. The first amalgam war raged between 1841 and 1855. The controversy was over the safety of mercury being used in dentistry. The society determined that mercury-silver fillings were unsafe and required a pledge from its members not to use amalgam because it was "unfit" to fill teeth.[22]

If a member did not sign this pledge, he or she would be expelled from the organization. Over time, most dentists voluntarily withdrew from the organization since they were using these new mercury-silver fillings.

When the American Society of Dental Surgeons held a meeting in 1856, there were not enough dentists present, and the society was disbanded for lack of a quorum. There were not enough dentists present to transact business legally.

With the demise of the American Society of Dental Surgeons, various state dental societies formed, which led to a national organization, the American Dental Association. The acceptance of dental amalgam was solid. The American Dental Association backed the safety of mercury-silver fillings; it was their defining issue. To this day, the American Dental Association insists that dental amalgams are safe despite increasing scientific and clinical evidence that they are *not* safe.

An amalgam is defined as a *mixture* of mercury with other metals. Generally, a mercury-silver filling is formed with approximately 50 percent mercury and a mixture of silver, copper, tin, and a small amount

---

[22] Bremner, *The Story of Dentistry*, 153.

of zinc. It is *not* a chemical compound, as some proponents of amalgam claim. Proponents of amalgam state that amalgam does not present the toxic danger that mercury does because of the mixing of mercury with other metals. They are wrong! Amalgam is an unstable *mixture* and not a stable alloy.

Mercury	50% *
Silver, tin, copper, zinc mixture	50% *

*Approximate

For many years, the "bread and butter" of dentistry has been fillings. "Drill and fill" took up a major part of a dentist's practice. If you had a cavity and went to a dentist, you had to expect to get a silver filling. The idea of a silver filling was so emphasized that even today, many people do not realize what a dental silver filling actually is.

Years ago, dentists made a silver filling by combining mercury and the silver and metal mixture powder with a mortar and pestle. After mixing the mercury and silver mixture, the dentist would place the mixture in a small cloth and squeeze out the excess mercury. Perhaps he didn't squeeze as much and more mercury was left in the mixture, a sobering thought for the patient receiving that silver filling! This process of mixing and inserting mercury-silver fillings exposes both the dentist and the patient to terrible mercury vapor.

As time went by, life got easier for dentists. They no longer had to manually mix mercury with the silver alloy. The amalgamator was invented. I remember using the Wigglebug, an early amalgamator, for many years. The dentist would place mercury and silver powder or pellets into a little black capsule. A metal ball would also be placed in this capsule. A top would be placed on the open capsule to keep the contents from spilling out. The capsule would then be placed in the metal arms of the amalgamator. The capsule would be shaken back and forth in the amalgamator, mixing the mercury and silver alloy. Many times, I would find little droplets of mercury around the machine as mercury would escape from the capsule during shaking. In the last few decades, most dentists have been using disposable pre-encapsulated alloy. At the factory, a sealed capsule containing mercury and the silver metal mixture is prepared. This is a convenience to the dentist since it saves him the time spent on the procedure of placing mercury and the silver mixture in the capsule. Most important of all, the capsule has very little mercury leakage upon mixing since it has a seal made at the factory. This exposes the dentist to less mercury vapor.

Dentist to patient: "Open wide!" Next comes the mercury-silver filling being pressed into your tooth cavity. You hear the metallic scrunch as the dentist presses the amalgam firmly into the tooth. You hear the metallic scraping off of the excess filling. Here, the dentist is carving the filling to a proper shape. The excess filling material is removed from your tooth. The dentist is taught to take excess scrap silver filling from your mouth and place it in a sealed jar covered with liquid. Is your mouth the only place where this mercury-silver filling is safe? If mercury is truly locked into the silver filling, why does the dentist have to be concerned about sealing it in a jar? This makes no consistent sense if mercury-silver fillings are safe in the mouth!

A good question is why a common dental filling is called a silver filling. Why not say a mercury-silver filling? Is there something about mercury that is so negative that it cannot be used in the name? Is it because it is a known poison? We have heard how dangerous a broken mercury thermometer is. So what about mercury in a dental filling?

Professor Alfred Stock, a leading German chemist, was instrumental in the second "amalgam war" regarding the safety of mercury in dentistry. This occurred around 1926 to 1932. It ended when his chemistry lab was destroyed by bombs dropped by the Allies during World War II.

In 1981, the Swedish neurobiologist Mats Hanson played a strong part in starting the third amalgam war. Dr. Huggins brought the issue of mercury leaking from dental fillings to the American public's attention. The amalgam wars were about the safety of mercury in dental fillings. Dr. Huggins received a lot of flak from established dentistry because of his position on amalgam.

It seems that throughout history, if a fact is not convenient, it is heresy. Remember Galileo saying the earth was round and revolved around the sun? Galileo was an Italian physicist and astronomer credited with building the first effective telescope. He used this to prove that the earth moves around the sun. This confirmed the theory originally put forward by the Polish astronomer Nicholas Copernicus. But it went directly against the teachings of the Church i.e.; the earth was the center of the Universe and the Sun revolved round the Earth. It was this conflict with the teachings of the Church that was to eventually bring Galileo to the attention of the Inquisition. According to the church, Galileo had committed heresy. History has a way of repeating itself.

Dr. Huggins was not the only dentist to be vocal about mercury in dentistry and to have suffered persecution from his state dental board because of it. There were others who were also persecuted for their concern, such as Dr. Joel Berger, who had a dental practice in New York. Dr. Berger was outspoken on the dental amalgam issue. Dr. Bob, a strong proponent of the safety of dental amalgam, was instrumental in Dr. Berger losing his license. There are other dentists who, with a good conscience to help their patients, ran into grief for presenting the truth about amalgams leaking mercury. By the way, this is the same Dr. Bob whom the insurance company used as an expert witness against me. He was a major factor in me losing my workers' compensation case.

The stand of the ADA is that dental amalgam is a safe restorative material. They claim that it has been used for over 150 years without incident and that for only a few who are allergic to amalgam is it a problem. They are profoundly wrong.

The following is the ADA's statement on mercury in dental amalgam: "Once mercury is combined with dental silver, its toxic properties are made inert." This statement still stands today, although there is strong scientific evidence contradicting the safety of dental amalgam.

Now, with advanced scientific methods that did not exist in the 1800s, let's explore mercury in today's common dental amalgam.

Mercury Droplets
Appear on silver filling[23]

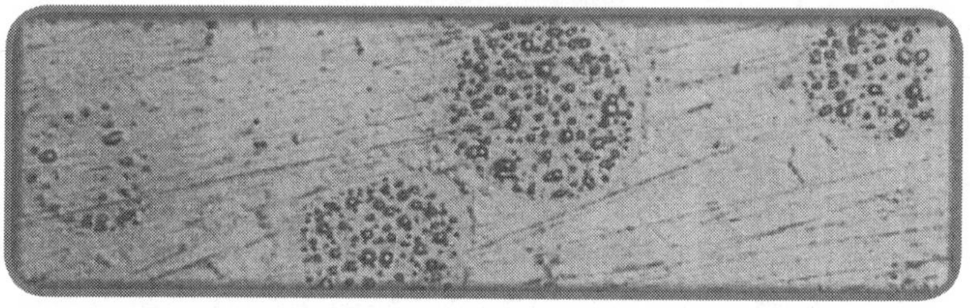

Photomicrograph (from Masi, 1994)

This is a photomicrograph of a mercury-silver filling taken with an electron microscope.[24] Minimal pressure was placed on several points of this twenty-five-year-old silver filling, which then showed mercury droplets. These are droplets of pure mercury just the same as you would find in a mercury thermometer. These droplets release mercury vapor, a very dangerous and toxic vapor, the kind that nearly killed me. Advocates of the safety of dental amalgam state that mercury is locked into the filling. Here, we see mercury as a separate entity from the silver powder it has been mixed with.

---

[23] Photo provided by IAOMT

[24] Masi, JV. Corrosion of Restorative Materials: The Problem and the Promise. Symposium: Status Quo and Perspectives of Amalgam and Other Dental Materials, April 29-May 1, (1994).

The Smoking Tooth[25]

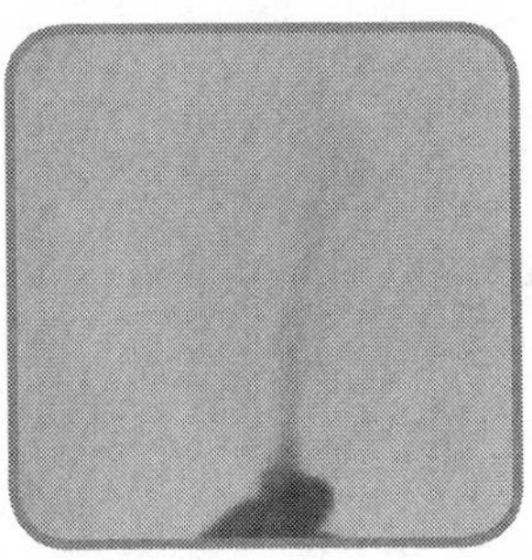

This is a photo of a 25 year old mercury-silver filling giving off mercury vapor. Mercury vapor is actually invisible to the human eye, but when ultraviolet light from the mercury vapor lamp is shined into a fluorescent screen, any mercury vapor that passes through that region will be selectively absorbed by the ultraviolet light, casting a shadow on the screen. We are seeing the evidence of the fact that mercury vapor "smokes" off of an amalgam's surface. Experiments can be performed to see what actions (rubbing, brushing, scraping) increase the release of mercury vapor from the surface of an amalgam. We find that rubbing an eraser against the silver filling increases the mercury vaporizing. Every time you drink a hot liquid or chew your food, mercury vapor release increases about tenfold. This measured result has been published in the scientific literature by Vimy, Lorscheider and others.

Video: http://iaomt.org/videos/
Presentation by David Kennedy, DDS

[25] Photo provided by IAOMT

Jerome Mercury Vapor Analyzer

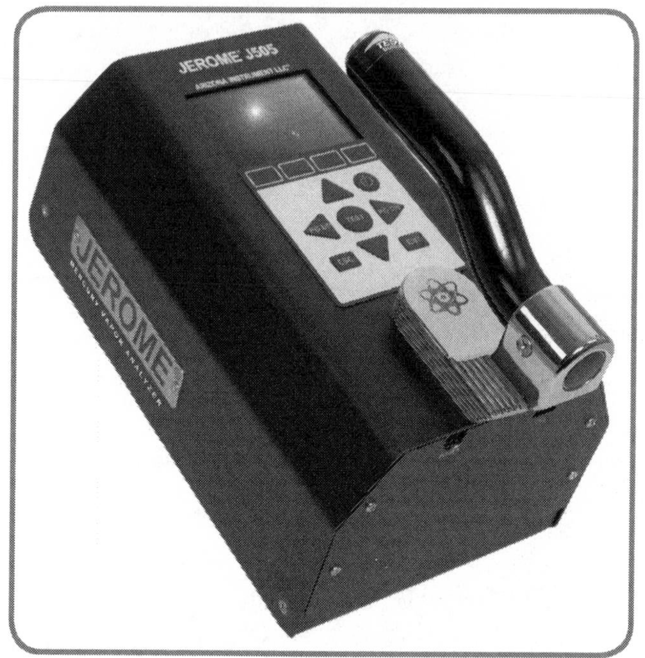

Extremely Accurate Device for Measuring Mercury Vapor

The Jerome Mercury Vapor Analyzer is manufactured by Arizona Instrument LLC. This device helped to fuel the third amalgam war.

When I first visited Dr. Michael Ziff in his office in Orlando, he demonstrated the Jerome Mercury Vapor Analyzer to me. He placed the probe over the amalgams in a patient's mouth. The device did not measure any mercury. Then he had the patient chew gum for a minute or two. He again placed the air intake probe over the patient's amalgams. The reading registered quite high. I saw for myself that mercury was being released. How stable is amalgam, then, if it is releasing mercury? No amount of mercury exposure can be considered safe. Jokingly, Dr. Ziff assured me it was mercury-free gum! Chewing or pressure against the patient's amalgams caused the release of mercury.

Regarding stability, when amalgam was first used to fill teeth, there was a serious problem. The amalgam expanded after a while and caused fracturing of the tooth. By later changing the proportion of the metals in the mixture, this problem was resolved. It is the proportions of silver, tin, copper, and zinc with respect to each other that makes the amalgam appear stable. An improper combination could cause either expansion or contraction of the amalgam. Stability is therefore only an illusion.

Sheep Study

Full-body scan of a sheep twenty-nine days after placement of twelve occlusal amalgams labeled with 203Hg. The fillings were removed prior to the scan:

In this famous animal study, mercury-silver fillings were placed in a sheep's teeth. The mercury used in these amalgams was chemically the same as any other mercury. But the nuclei in the atoms of this mercury were radioactive, meaning, the mercury gave off radiation that could be measured. In just thirty days, mercury spread from the teeth to the jawbone, the kidneys, the heart, and the hoof. All the teeth with amalgams had been removed prior to this scan. Therefore, only mercury transferred to the body of the sheep would be detected. The mercury in the jaw was significant as the mercury spread from the fillings to the jawbone.[26]

Advocates of mercury use in fillings claimed that sheep chew too much. The ADA and the amalgam defenders dismissed the study's relevance to human's use of dental amalgam because sheep spend much more time chewing than humans do.

Monkey Study

A full body scan was performed on a monkey showing distribution of mercury. The scan indicated a similar spread of mercury throughout

---

[26] Hahn, LJ; Kloiber, R; Leininger, RW; Vimy, MJ; Lorscheider, FL. Dental "silver" tooth fillings: a source of mercury exposure revealed by whole body scan and tissue analysis. FASEB J, 3:2641-6, 1989.

the monkey body. Monkeys have a similar chewing pattern to humans. So the critics of the sheep study are wrong.[27]

Then how about humans? Would we not accumulate mercury from mercury-silver fillings too?

[27] Hahn, LJ; et al. Whole-Body Imaging of the Distribution of Mercury Released from Dental Fillings into Monkey Tissues. FASEB J. 4:3256-609 1990.

Graphic Representation of the Distribution of Mercury in a Human From Dental Amalgams

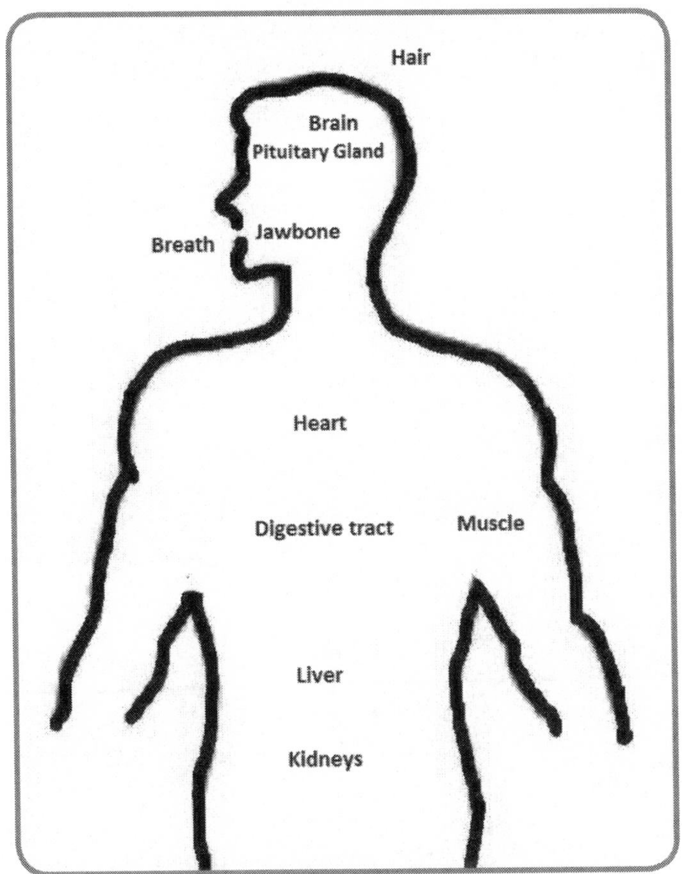

References for the Preceding Graphic

Breath

- Alfred Stock, Zeitschrift fuer angewandte Chemie, 29. Jahrgang, 15. April 1926, Nr. 15, S. 461-466, Die Gefaehrlichkeit des Quecksilberdampfes, von Alfred Stock (1926) The Dangerousness of Mercury Vapor

- Svare CW, Peterson LC, Reinhardt JW, Boyer DB, Frank CW, Gay DD, Cox RD: The effect of Dental Amalgams on mercury levels in expired air. J Dent Res. 60:1668-71, 1981
- Vimy MJ, Lorscheider FL: Intra-oral air mercury released from dental amalgam. J Den Res 64:1069-71, 1985

Hair

- Nixon GS, Smith H: Mercury hazards in dental surgeries. J Dent Res 43 Supplement to No. 5:968 (Abstract #63), 1964
- Amy S. Holmes, Mark F. Blaxill, Boyd E. Haley Reduced Levels of Mercury in First Baby Haircut of Autistic Children, International Journal of Toxicology 22:277-285, 2003

Brain

- D. W. Eggleston and M. Nylander, "Correlation of Dental Amalgam with Mercury in Brain Tissue," Journal of Prosthetic Dentistry 58 (1987): 704–707.

Hair, Blood, Brain, Toenail, Muscle

- Björkman L, Lundekvam BF, Laegreid T, Bertelsen BI, Morild I, Lilleng P, Lind B, Palm B, Vahter M, Environ Health. 2007 Oct 11;6:30.
- Mercury in human brain, blood, muscle and toenails in relation to exposure: an autopsy study. 2007 http://www.ehjournal.net/content/6/1/30

Brain, Kidney, Liver

- Drasch G, Schupp I, Riedl G, Gunter G. Einfluss von Amalgamfullungen auf die Quecksilberkonzentration in menschlichen Organen. Dtsch Zahn=E4rztl Z 47:490-496 (1992)

Milk

- Fujita, M. & Takabatake, E. T., Mercury Levels in Human Maternal and Neonate Blood, Hair and milk; Bull Environ Contam Toxicol., 18 (205-209) 1977
- Vol. X #17. Vimy, M.J., et.al., Mercury from Maternal "Silver" Tooth Fillings in Sheep and Human Breast Milk, Biological Trace Element Research, v.56 (1997). [vol. 10, no.14]
- Elaheh Norouzi · Nader Bahramifar · Seyed Mahmoud Ghasempouri, Effect of teeth amalgam on mercury levels in the colostrums human milk in Lenjan Environ Monit Assess 2011 DOI 10.1007/s10661-011-1974-1

Heart

- **IDCM:** Idiopathic Dilated Cardiomyopathy the most common reason for anyone in the US to need a heart transplant. Frustachi found 22,000 TIMES more mercury in hearts that died of IDCM than in hearts that died of heart attack.[28]

Women of childbearing age

Exposure of childbearing-aged women is of particular concern because of the potential adverse neurologic effects of Hg in fetuses. All women and children in the 1999--2002 NHANES survey period had blood Hg levels below 58 μg/L. The harm to a fetus from levels of exposure as measured by cord blood levels between 5.8 μg/L and 58 μg/L is uncertain. [29]

[28] Andrea Frustaci, MD, et. al., Marked elevation of myocardial trace elements in idiopathic dilated cardiomyopathy compared with secondary cardiac dysfunction, J Am Coll Cardiol, 1999; 33:1578-1583

[29] MMWR, Weekly, Mercury Levels in Young Children and Childbearing-Aged Women---United States, November 5, 2004 / 53(43);1018-1020

Kidney

- Mortada WL, Sobh MA, El-Defrawy MM, Farahat SE. Urology and Nephrology Center, Mansoura University, Faculty of Science, Egypt. J Nephrol 2002 Mar-Apr;15(2):171-6.

Urine

- Frykholm KO: On mercury from dental amalgam. Its toxic and allergic effects and some comments on occupational hygiene. Acta Odont Scand 15:7-108, suppl 22, 1957
- Fetus Drasch G, Schupp I, H=F6fl H, Reinke R & Roider G. Mercury burden of human fetal and infant tissues. Eur J Pediatr 153:607-610 (1994)

Tooth roots and in Jaw bones

- Till, T., Maaly, K. Mercury in tooth roots and in Jaw bones. Zahnarztl Welt/Reform (ZWR) Vol 87 Issue 6 Pg 288-90 1978
- Hahn, Leszek J.; Kloiber, Reinhard; Leininger, Ronald W.; Vimy, Murray J.; & Lorscheider, Fritz L.
- Whole-body imaging of the distribution of mercury released from dental fillings into monkey tissues. FASEB, Vol. 4, Nov. 1990, pp. 3256-3260.

Jawbone, Kidneys, Gastrointestinal Tract, Heart

- Hahn, LJ; et al. Whole-Body Imaging of the Distribution of Mercury Released from Dental Fillings into Monkey Tissues. FASEB J. 4:3256-609 1990.
- Hahn, LJ; Kloiber, R; Leininger, RW; Vimy, MJ; Lorscheider, FL. Dental "silver" tooth fillings: a source of mercury exposure revealed by whole body scan and tissue analysis. FASEB J, 3:2641-6, 1989.

At a Los Angeles coroner's office, accident victims of sudden death, as from an auto accident, were used in a study. The numbers of occlusal fillings were counted. A test to determine the concentration of mercury in brain tissue was performed. The results were that there was a direct correlation between the amount of mercury-silver fillings and the concentration of mercury in brain tissue.

> "Data from this project demonstrate a positive correlation between the number of occlusal surfaces of dental amalgam and mercury levels in the brain."[30]

In another document, mercury exposure from amalgams is again corroborated:

As Guzzi explained in a research paper in 2006, the amount of mercury released from dental amalgam is significant.[31]

There is variability on the release of mercury from an amalgam. Brushing, chewing, and drinking hot liquids can increase the amount of mercury emitted. In addition, various brands of amalgams emit different amounts of mercury. The way a dentist mixes amalgam can be a factor. The use of pre-encapsulated alloy has standardized the amount of mercury in an amalgam. However, trituration (mixing) time varies and can affect how well the mercury and the silver alloy are combined.

> "In a study of long term dissolution of mercury from a supposedly non-mercury releasing amalgam, it was determined that 43.5 microgram/cm2/day Hg was released and this remained constant for 2 years."[32]

> "Thus, the previously reported 43.5 micrograms/cm2/day and the values found in the IAOMT amalgam studies are not an insignificant amount of mercury exposure when

---

30 D. W. Eggleston and M. Nylander, "Correlation of Dental Amalgam with Mercury in Brain Tissue," *Journal of Prosthetic Dentistry* 58 (1987): 704–707.

31 G. Guzzi et al., "Dental Amalgam and Mercury Levels in Autopsy Tissues: Food for Thought," *American Journal of Forensic Medicine and Pathology* 27, no. 1 (2006) 42–45.

32 Chew et al., "Long-Term Dissolution of Mercury from a Non-Mercury-Releasing Amalgam," *Clinical Preventive Dentistry* 13, no. 3 (1991): 5–7.

> one considers the number of years a 70-year old individual living today may have been exposed to chronic mercury levels from his or her amalgam fillings. Additionally, this release per day is the level released without *galvanism* (electric currents), excess heat, or pressure from chewing—all factors that increase mercury release from amalgams in the mouth." "Some may disagree with the preceding (high) mercury emission values . . . However, even the lowest values we report represent toxic exposures."[33]
>
> "Also, the World Health Organization Scientific Panel found ranges of mercury exposures from 3 to 70 micrograms/day, with the bulk being from amalgam fillings."[34]

The current Occupational Safety and Health Administration (OSHA) permissible exposure limit (PEL) for mercury vapor is 0.1 milligram per cubic meter of air as a ceiling limit. A worker's exposure to mercury vapor should, at no time, exceed this ceiling level.

The advocates of silver-mercury fillings justify the safety of mercury by using urine and blood mercury levels. These levels may vary during different times. Furthermore, these levels do not account for tissue absorption and excretion through the feces. "First, it is well known that about 85 to 95% of mercury is excreted in the feces and not the urine, so why perform estimates based on urinary mercury levels?"

The use of urine mercury levels of people who are poor excretors would suggest that they have not been exposed to much mercury. However, the mercury in their tissues may be quite high. Mercury hair levels also may be misleading: "High hair-mercury levels indicate the ability to excrete and low hair-mercury levels indicate an impaired ability to excrete."

---

[33] B. E. Haley, "The Relationship of the Toxic Effects of Mercury to Exacerbation of the Medical Condition Classified as Alzheimer's Disease," *Medical Veritas* 4 (2007): 1514–1515.

[34] FDA Presentation: An Evaluation of Dental Amalgam Mercury Release and Corresponding Toxicology Concerns, by Boyd E. Haley, PhD, professor, Department of Chemistry, University of Kentucky (September 7, 2006), 1.

The body's exposure to mercury over time is cumulative dependent on how efficiently it can eliminate the poison. In addition, as a person gets older, he or she can become less efficient in removing mercury as certain enzyme and detoxification systems break down with age.

It just shows that most physicians have been looking at this incorrectly. There is science pointing to mercury as a probable cause of or contributing factor in all such chronic neurological and autoimmune illnesses. This includes Alzheimer's disease (AD), autism, ALS, MS, and Parkinson's disease.[35] This hypothesis is dismissed by major research programs, although mercury, the most neurotoxic metal in mercury-silver fillings, is just inches away from the brain. Although mercury from dental amalgam is listed as a source of toxicity, it is just ignored. The following video is compelling regarding mercury and AD:

Do a Google search as the address for this video may change: "How Mercury Destroys the Brain - University of Calgary"

Researcher David Eggleston, DDS, also did a study on the effects of dental amalgams and dental nickel alloy on T-lymphocytes. These white blood cells play an important part in immunity.

> "An abnormal T-lymphocyte percent of lymphocytes can increase the risk of cancer, infectious diseases, and autoimmune disease.
>
> Preliminary data suggest that dental amalgam and dental nickel alloys can adversely affect the quantity of T-lymphocytes."[36]

On the subject of galvanism, it is very easy to measure the electric currents in the mouth. When metals are in the mouth, they produce

---

[35] B. E. Haley, "The Relationship of the Toxic Effects of Mercury to Exacerbation of the Medical Condition Classified as Alzheimer's Disease," *Medical Veritas* 4 (2007): 1510–1524.

[36] David Eggleston, "Effect of Dental Amalgam and Nickel Alloys on T-Lymphocytes: Preliminary Report," *Journal of Prosthetic Dentistry* 31, no. 5 (May 1984).

a "battery effect," and this battery is capable of producing electric currents that flow between the different metal surfaces in the mouth. The mouth is like a battery. You have saliva, which acts as an electrolyte (conducts electricity), and various metals with different electromotive potentials, which produce an electric voltage. I have personally seen mercury-silver fillings with very high levels of current measured in microamperes. When the current flows more strongly, as when gold crowns are added to a mouth that already has amalgams, more mercury is released from the amalgam surfaces.

The American Dental Association reaffirmed the safety of dental amalgam. However, in contrast to this statement of safety, the following is the legal position of the ADA:

> "The ADA owes *no legal duty of care to protect the public* from allegedly dangerous products used by dentists. The ADA did not manufacture, design, supply or install the mercury-containing amalgams. The ADA does not control those who do. The ADA's only alleged involvement in the product was to provide information regarding its use. Dissemination of information relating to the practice of dentistry does not create a duty of care to protect the public from potential injury."

The source of the above statement is the legal brief filed in 1995 by the attorneys of the ADA in *W. H. Tolhurst v. Johnson and Johnson Consumer Products, Inc.; Engelhard Corporation; ABE Dental, Inc.; the American Dental Association, et al.*, in the Superior Court of the State of California, in and for the County of Santa Clara, California, case number 718228.

This statement is a call to dentists still using amalgam: dentists may not have the American Dental Association's backing should there be a lawsuit on damage from mercury-silver fillings.

Chapter 22

About Mercury

Leading Sources of Mercury Pollution in Washington State

Source: Washington Department of Ecology

Mercury builds up in the environment, where concentrations increase as they move up the food chain. Dentists are among the largest users of the toxic substance - in amalgam fillings.

Leading sources of mercury pollution in pounds per year:

Products containing mercury: 1,898
Gold mining: 777
Coal-fired power plants.................................. 436
Manufacturing:.. 296

Breakdown of products containing mercury in pounds per year at time of disposal

Fluorescent lamps.. 507
Thermostats 431
Dental amalgam from dental facilities............ 404
Auto convenience light switches 219

Dental amalgam in feces and urine..................62
Household fever thermometers..........................12

Contribution to the body burden of mercury from the World Health Organization (WHO) 1991 approximate

Dental Amalgam.. 17 micrograms/day
Seafood.. 2 micrograms/day

Another deadly insidious source of mercury is from the use of Thimerosal. Thimerosal is a deadly mercury compound that should be banned completely. It is used as a preservative in various vaccines that come in multi-dose vials.

Symptoms of Mercury Poisoning[37]

- *Behavioral.* Depression, emotional instability (mood swings), inability to concentrate, sleep disturbances, irritability, and forgetfulness.
- *Cardiovascular.* Abnormal heartbeat, pressure and pain in chest, high or low blood pressure, and anemia. Mercury can damage blood vessels, reducing blood supply to the tissues. Heart problems have been reported.
- *Blood.* Adverse effects on red blood cells. Mercury binds to hemoglobin in the red blood cells, thus reducing oxygen-carrying capacity.
- *Central nervous system.* Light and sound sensitivity, headaches, convulsions, tremors, muscle twitches, numbness and tingling of the extremities, dizziness, hearing or vision difficulty, and black-and-white dreams (instead of colored).
- *Detoxification systems.* By overloading the detoxification pathways, other toxins are eliminated less efficiently.
- *Digestive.* Constipation or diarrhea (alternating), digestion problems, colitis, loss of appetite, ulcers, bloating and gas, and loss of smell and taste.

[37] *William R. Kellas, PhD and Andrea Sharon Dworkin, N.D., "Surviving the Toxic Crisis", 1996, Page 187-188.*

- *Endocrine.* Thyroid dysfunction, low body temperature, cold hands and feet, decreased libido, frequent night urination, leg and muscle cramps, joint pain, kidney stones, and slow healing.
- *Energy.* Chronic fatigue, drowsiness, hypoglycemia, and muscle weakness.
- *Immune system.* Allergies, asthma, environmental illness, Hodgkin's disease, swollen glands, and susceptibility to colds and infection.
- *Joints and muscles.* Arthritis, fibromyalgia, and lupus.
- *Kidney problems.*
- *Oral cavity.* Bad breath, bleeding gums, canker sores, bone loss, increased salivation (due to battery effect), metallic taste, periodontal (gum and jawbone) disease, purple black pigment in gum adjacent to a silver filling (sometimes called mercury tattoo), leukoplakia (an oral precancerous condition caused by local metal irritation).
- *Reproductive.* Infertility, miscarriage, and premature birth.
- *Skin.* Acne, itching, skin flushing, rough skin, and rashes.

Mercury: Influences on Body Chemistry

Reproductive effects. Infertility, miscarriage, and premature birth. Mercury lowers the levels of progesterone, which is needed to allow the uterus to support pregnancy. Progesterone insufficiency may be associated with low libido (sex drive) and premenstrual syndrome (PMS). Low progesterone levels can lead to infertility. In fact, PMS and infertility are common among young female dental workers due at least in part to their mercury exposure.

Male dental workers also have a relatively high incidence of infertility. Mercury also leads to lower testosterone (male hormone) levels. Both progesterone and testosterone productions are zinc dependent. Mercury interferes with zinc metabolism and thereby indirectly affects hormone production.

Mineral displacement. Mercury (usually with a +2 charge) can grab the biological spaces that should be filled by another essential mineral. As a result, there may be plenty of the mineral in the blood, urine, hair, etc.; but because of the displacement at the active site, mercury interferes with the activity of the essential mineral.

Symptoms that may be caused by minerals depleted by mercury include the following:

- *Magnesium.* Irregular heartbeat, chocolate cravings, cramps, PMS, receding gums, elevated blood pressure, etc.
- *Iron.* Anemia, fatigue, etc.
- *Copper.* Anemia, thyroid dysfunction, impaired digestion, problems with liver enzymes (which are all copper dependent), easy bruising, etc.
- *Zinc.* Anorexia nervosa, loss of taste and smell, loss of appetite, low libido, PMS, impaired growth, acne and other skin disorders, etc.
- *Iodine.* Thyroid dysfunction, thickened bile, etc.

Digestive effects. Mercury acts as an antibacterial and has been used in some medicines (vaccines, eye drops, etc.). It can be an important cause of bowel yeast or parasite overgrowth and harmful organisms because it kills off beneficial bacteria, which normally repel parasites and aid digestion. Yeast overgrowth—with its attendant symptoms of fatigue, brain fog, sweets cravings, and vaginal yeast infections—is often traced to the antibiotic effect of dental mercury. Suspect this as a root cause when yeast is a continuing problem in spite of repeated treatment. The symptom (yeast overgrowth) will not likely go away until the root cause (mercury) is dealt with. The effect of dental mercury on normal gut flora is well documented.

Thyroid problems. These problems, such as low body temperature, often improve when mercury-containing amalgams are removed. Normal body temperature, measured orally, is about 98.6 degrees Fahrenheit. Those with a temperature range of 96.2 to 97.6 degrees are often considered to have hypothyroidism (low thyroid function). It has been observed that their temperature can rise to 98.2 in as little as one day after amalgam removal and to 98.6 soon afterward. It is plausible that a low body temperature, which can be a sign of low thyroid function, is another symptom caused by mercury. Of course, it would be far better to correct the cause of the apparent thyroid malfunction by removing the fillings or other causes responsible for lower body temperature, rather than just prescribing thyroid hormone.

Brain and learning. Brain defects and learning disabilities present at birth can be caused by mercury, as the metal can pass through both the placental barrier and the blood-brain barrier to the fetus. There is a sheep study documenting that the fetus accumulates and concentrates the mercury from the mother!

Accumulation in the brain leads to mental and nervous system problems, such as brain fog, depression, vision difficulties, and others listed above. Mental effects are among the most common due to mercury's strong affinity for the brain. Mercury inhibits the effects of certain neurotransmitters:

- *Dopamine.* Pain control and well-being
- *Serotonin.* Relaxation, sleep, and well-being
- *Adrenaline.* Energy and stamina
- *Noradrenalin and melatonin.* Sleep cycles

Mercury's inhibition of these neurotransmitters can account in part for the feelings of depression and loss of motivation.

Other mental and/or neurological symptoms are the following:

- General neurological symptoms
- Mental illness
- Demyelinization, which can lead to such diseases as multiple sclerosis
- Developmental problems
- Cerebral palsy
- ALS (amyotrophic lateral sclerosis, or Lou Gehrig's disease)
- Alzheimer's disease
- Psychological problems, including loss of function and memory, anger and emotionality, and timidity

Mercury effect on energy. Mercury binds to sulfur in proteins, oxygen from the lungs, sulfur from the liver's detoxification systems, and selenium from the colon. Lower levels of body tissue oxygen because of mercury's binding to it may lead to the following:

- There is fatigue caused by low blood sugar, secondary to low blood oxygen.
- Parasite infestation results from an anaerobic (less oxygen) environment and low levels of the good bacteria, which fight off parasites.
- An anaerobic environment also favors the development of yeast infections and cancer since yeast is a fermenting spore and cancer is a fermenting cell, rather than a normal respiratory (oxygen using) cell.
- Mercury binds with hemoglobin, which is located inside the red blood cell and carries oxygen to tissues. Mercury bound to hemoglobin results in less oxygen-carrying capacity of the red blood cell, and as a result, less oxygen reaches the tissues. The body senses the need for more oxygen and may attempt to compensate by increasing the production of hemoglobin. A normal or increased hemoglobin level combined with symptoms of lack of oxygen (fatigue, weakness, paleness, rapid heart rate, shortness of breath, etc.) could indicate mercury toxicity. This can confuse the doctor since the patient seems anemic but the blood counts seem fine.
- Copper is also required to prevent anemia, and mercury can compete for copper's binding sites. In this case, a low hematocrit (red blood cell count) can be indicative of low blood copper levels.
- The terms *hematocrit* and *hemoglobin*, routinely found on blood test printouts, can be confusing. If blood were likened to a train carrying oxygen to where it is needed, hematocrit would be the boxcars on the train (red blood cells), while hemoglobin would be the carrying capacity of each boxcar, or red blood cell. When there is low hematocrit (less boxcars), the condition is called anemia.
- The activity of other minerals on metabolism and energy production can be reduced by mercury's tendency to fight for

the site. An inefficiency in the functioning of minerals can lead to fatigue and other symptoms:

1. Cobalt, calcium, magnesium, potassium, and sodium are all required for energy.
2. Zinc is needed for the manufacture of adrenaline.
3. Cobalt, a component of vitamin B12, prevents pernicious anemia, which can cause fatigue.
4. Mercury blocks magnesium and manganese transport required for memory functioning, resulting in decreased ability to concentrate.

These mineral deficiencies may be primarily due to dietary deficiencies. However, deficiencies may also be caused by mercury poisoning. The mineral may be in the body but cannot get to where it is needed because mercury has blocked the way. Lab tests can only tell the mineral levels available—they do not tell if the minerals are performing their functions in the body. Symptoms and physical signs often help dispel the illusion that the "lab results are all normal."

Increased toxicity. The mercuric ion (Hg^{+2}) binds to sulfhydryl groups (-SH) in proteins and disulfide groups (-SS) in amino acids. These sulfur-containing groups have an important detoxification function in the body by binding to a variety of chemicals, toxins, minerals, etc. When mercury binds to these sulfur groups, the ability to detoxify chemicals decreases.

When mercury binds the bile, the ability of the body to absorb fat decreases, leading to increased absorption of toxic oil-soluble chemicals, such as solvents and pesticides, like a dry sponge.

Selenium is an antioxidant that protects against free radical damage from chemicals, which can lead to cancer. Mercury can bind to selenium, making this protective mechanism useless.

What else can mercury do?[38]

---

[38] *William R. Kellas, PhD and Andrea Sharon Dworkin, N.D,. "Surviving the Toxic Crisis", 1996, Page 193.*

Mercurous ion (Hg^{+1}) pushes out Na^{+1} (sodium), K^{+1} (potassium), and Li^{+1} (lithium). Sodium and potassium are part of the cellular sodium-potassium pump, which causes muscle movement. Interference with sodium and potassium can lead to muscle weakness for this reason. Leg and muscle cramps may be due to potassium deficiency.

Lithium is sometimes given as lithium carbonate to patients suffering from bipolar depression (manic-depressive illness) since lack of lithium is one of the causes of the disease. Lack of lithium may itself be caused by mercury preventing lithium from working as it should in the brain. Therefore, mercury may cause depression by reducing lithium.

Mercury is like a two-hundred-pound bully attacking a seven-pound baby; the small baby doesn't have much of a chance. Two hundred is the molecular weight of mercury (the bully) and 7 is the molecular weight of lithium (the baby). If you have been diagnosed with bipolar depression, maybe you need less mercury, not more lithium pills.

Mercury fights for binding sites in the kidney, another organ to which it has a special affinity. A mineral and electrolyte balance are needed in order for the kidney to perform its functions, and a poorly functioning kidney can lead to edema (fluid buildup in the body). These minerals are prevented from entering into their reactions when mercury interferes. Suppression of potassium by mercury also affects the kidneys, which takes you from making adrenaline to maintaining electrolyte balance, and the low adrenaline level can lead to low energy.

Detoxification systems, such as metallothionein, cytochrome P-450, and bile, are adversely affected by mercury. Metallothionein binds toxic metals in the body to prepare them for excretion. Mercury ties up this material so it cannot clear out other metals, such as lead, cadmium, and aluminum.

Mercury from amalgam binds to -SH (sulfhydryl) groups, which are used in almost every enzymatic process in the body. It therefore has the potential to disturb all metabolic processes.

Some people seem allergic to whatever food they eat. No matter what they eat, at least one thing is constantly ingested: mercury (or nickel).

Mercury released from amalgam during chewing may be the cause of most of the symptoms that seem to be caused by the food. If a mercury vapor test is done, it may show a low to moderate level of mercury initially but a sharply increased level after chewing gum. This is also what happens when food is chewed. Such a test result, combined with apparent allergy to most food, points to mercury as a probable culprit. Nickel, which may also be contributing to the problem, is in stainless steel dental posts and braces.[39] Nickel has also been used in crowns and as a metal base for porcelain crowns

Another neurotransmitter that mercury can block is GABA. Low GABA can be related to anxiety conditions. Valium is used in combination with a psychotropic drug to raise GABA levels. It is best to have a physician prescribe a therapy and not self-medicate. All psychotropic drugs have their potential toxicities, so it is advisable to use other methods to optimize neurotransmitters. Detoxification, the use of minerals, amino acids, and diet may be useful.[40]

Mercury has a great affinity for sulfide bonds, which means it likes kidneys, livers, red blood cells, and the central nervous system.[41]

Mercury affects fetal formation.[42]

In the book, "Evidence of Harm", David Kirby writes about mercury in vaccines and the autism epidemic. Thimerosal is a mercury compound that is used as a preservative in multi-vial doses for vaccinations. This was used in childhood vaccines.

There is no question in my mind that thimerosal in these vaccines damages babies. At the age of 3 months, my son was given his vaccinations which contained thimerosal. He had an immediate adverse reaction. That very

---

39 *William R. Kellas, PhD and Andrea Sharon Dworkin, N.D., "Surviving the Toxic Crisis", 1996, above paraphrased: 181-211.*

40 The San Francisco Medical Research Foundation, http://www.lightparty.com/Health/Anxiety.html.

41 *American Journal of Physiology*, 261, no. 30 (1991): R1010–R1014.

42 *British Medical Journal* 32, no. 1 (1976), and *Environmental Health Perspective* 108, no. 3 (2000): 373–374.

first night, he cried hysterically. Prior to this, he slept well. After this, for the next 6 months, he cried at night. He developed a dark black line under both his eyes. His development was slow. He was refused at a pre-kindergarten school as they said, "your son has a neurological disorder". He had to go to special education class for a learning language disability. Can you imagine the suffering a child sustains if he reacts to the thimerosal in a vaccine. The developing brain is very susceptible to the damage done by mercury. The disability incurred may last the rest of the child's life. Fortunately, thimerosal is no longer used in childhood vaccinations. However, it is still used in flu shots.

A reason given for autism is the inability to detoxify mercury. In children having ASD (autism spectrum disorder), the ratio was 80 percent boys and 20 percent girls. The higher rate of autism in boys was attributed to testosterone suppressing MT (metallothionein), while estrogen enhances it. MT functions with its chemical cousin glutathione to bind with mercury and other heavy metals.[43]

In personal communication with Dr. Boyd Haley, he states: "I know of nothing that increases the toxicity of mercury or ethylmercury to a greater degree than testosterone. In contrast, estradiol gave protective results against thimerosal toxicity to neurons." In scientific research, it was found that the addition of testosterone to thimerosal greatly increased neuron death.[44]

Mercury alters gastrointestinal tract bacteria, which affects digestion.[45]

Mercury is capable of inducing autoimmune diseases.[46] Mercury can cause people to be at risk for lower fertility.[47]

---

[43] David Kirby, "Evidence of Harm", (2005), 144.

[44] B.E. Haley, Mercury toxicity: "Genetic susceptibility and synergistic effects", Medical Veritas 2 (2005) 537.

[45] *Antimicrobial Agents and Chemotherapy* (April 1993), 825–834.

[46] McCann and Scheckner, "Hyperthyroidism Associated with Mercury Poisoning," 742–743.

[47] *Journal of Toxicology and Environmental Health,* part A, no. 54 (1998): 593–611.

I have included the following on the adrenal gland as a possible cause of fatigue. Millions of people suffer from exhaustion. Many have chronic fatigue syndrome. The adrenal glands sit on top of the kidneys. Dehydroepiandrosterone (DHEA) is a steroid hormone that is mainly secreted by the adrenal glands. It serves as a precursor to other hormones, such as testosterone, androstenedione, and estrogen. DHEA has many functions. It seems to be associated with energy and immunity. Mercury can accumulate in the adrenal glands and cause them to become dysfunctional. Heavy metals, such as mercury, and stress can cause adrenal burnout. This, in turn, can cause fatigue and a decreased ability to cope with stress. A physician can test for DHEA levels to see if there is a connection to fatigue. Removing mercury from the body and adrenal nutritional support is a treatment option. DHEA supplementation under the monitoring of a physician may also be helpful.

Mercury is capable of altering DNA within any cell. Mercury ions, once in the body, combine with a methyl ion, resulting in a new compound, methylmercury, which is a hundred times more toxic than a mercury ion alone. Mercury affects and/or destroys any and all cells it comes in contact with. Some of the diseases and conditions that may be caused by mercury exposure are chronic fatigue syndrome, lupus, insomnia, memory loss, seizures, sinus problems, rashes, immunosuppression, chemical sensitivities, maldigestion, and many others.

In my research, trying to find out what happened to me, I came across a scientist who was researching the Gulf War syndrome. I sent Dr. Alan* a blood sample. I received an e-mail from him, stating, "Stu—we got something. We had to turn to a purely research test but we got results. It's just research, a hunch and lots of other disclaimers, okay?" The technique used was a PCR (polymerase chain reaction) test. The results were that they found that the RNA (ribonucleic acid) sequencing in plasma was pathological. The hot spot was chromosome 22q11.2. I contacted another mercury toxic dentist, Dr. Greg*, to have the same test performed. The results were identical to mine. Although this test was only in the initial research stage, this is further proof that mercury can alter cell function. Dr. Alan found that many of the victims of the Gulf War syndrome had similar alterations in their RNA sequencing pattern. This type of effect of mercury on the body makes me think about the statement that Dr. Friedmann's associate once told me: "Mercury in the body is like putting sand in a finely tuned watch."

DNA carries the genetic information of a cell and consists of thousands of genes. Each gene serves as a recipe on how to build a protein molecule. This information is then transmitted to the RNA to carry out these instructions. Proteins perform important tasks for cell functions or serve as building blocks. The information from the genes determines the protein composition and thereby the functions of the cell. The significance of this is that mercury can change protein formation within the cell and therefore the structure and function of the cell.

The combined effect of mercury and another toxic agent is extremely more toxic than mercury alone. "A dose of mercury sufficient to kill 1% of tested rats, when combined with a dose of lead sufficient to kill less than 1% of rats, resulted in killing 100% of rats tested."[48]

Toxic synergism: The synergistic effect of mercury with another toxic material is extremely much greater than the two of them individually. (Synergism is the interaction of elements that, when combined, produce a total effect that is greater than the sum of the individual elements.) Therefore, if you combine mercury in the body with aluminum, pesticides, tobacco smoke, cadmium, arsenic, etc., the effect can be devastating. This synergistic effect could play a part in multiple chemical sensitivity, where a person becomes extremely sensitive to chemicals in the environment.

Please refer to the following excellent sources of information on mercury:

- DAMS Fact Sheet, Dental Amalgam Fillings Are the Number One Source of Mercury in People and Exposures from Amalgam

---

[48] J. Schubert, E. J. Riley, and S. A. Tyler, "Combined Effects in Toxicology—a Rapid Systematic Testing Procedure: Cadmium, Mercury, and Lead," *Toxicol Environ Health* 4, nos. 5–6 (1978): 763–776.

Commonly Exceed Government Health Guidelines" (www.flcv.com/damspr1.html)
- Bernie Windham, Mechanisms by which mercury causes over 30 chronic health conditions (over 3,500 peer-reviewed studies), 2002 (www.flcv.com/indexa.html)

With all the information on mercury poisoning, why is it that you don't hear of anyone being poisoned by mercury with the above credible documentation?

A physician makes an initial differential diagnosis. Then he rules out possibilities with testing, etc. However, it is almost impossible to rule out mercury as a causative agent. Any exposure would make this cause a possibility. Mercury exposure can come from various sources, including mercury-silver fillings, occupational exposure, consumption of fish with high mercury levels, vaccinations (flu shots and others), and environmental exposure, such as being near a coal burning plant, a crematorium, etc. Mercury-silver fillings are responsible for the primary burden of mercury in the body. It is also possible for the fetus to accumulate maternal mercury. Some of the body burden of mercury in the mother can be passed on to the developing fetus.

In a study titled "10 Americans," cord blood from ten randomly selected babies across the country was analyzed. A total of 287 chemicals was found, including mercury. Babies are born pre-polluted. These chemicals are coming from the mother while she is pregnant. During pregnancy, the blood-brain barrier of the fetus is not fully developed, and pollutants can get into the developing brain. "The combined evidence suggests that neuro-developmental disorders caused by industrial chemicals has created a silent pandemic in modern society." For a video presentation on "10 Americans" by the Environmental Work Group (www.ewg.org), please google: "10 Americans Video".

The President's Council considers this pre-polluted contamination important:

> "Ideally, both mothers and fathers should avoid exposure to endocrine-disrupting chemicals and known or suspected carcinogens prior to child's conception and

> throughout pregnancy and early life, when risk of damage is greatest."[49]

The mercury challenge test has been used to determine a body burden. DMPS and DMSA have been used. These chemicals bind with mercury and help excrete mercury out of the body. Usually, a pre-challenge urine mercury level is performed. Then, subsequent to the administration of the chelating drug, another urine mercury level is taken. Increase of mercury in the urine is proof of a body burden. Yet there is no way of knowing how much mercury is stored in the body and how much damage it is causing. I was told about a physician who was so determined to find mercury in a patient that he administered twenty-five chelations. On the twenty-fifth chelation, the patient got sick and excreted a high amount of mercury. A positive test, therefore, is meaningful, but a negative test does not rule out mercury. DMPS and DMSA are not without hazards. Many chelators can cause a redistribution of toxins and an exacerbation of poisoning. Chelation challenge testing can make you sicker! Some people are at risk. I know because when I received the IV vitamin C and the IV EDTA, my symptoms were frightening following the procedure because I was so toxic.

Aside from chelating agents, which increase excretion of mercury, there are several other tests that look indirectly at the effects of mercury on the body.

Such a test is the porphyrin profile. This test was developed by Professor James S. Woods, PhD, at the University of Washington. He is the main inventor of the porphyrin test for mercury. Instead of looking for mercury, this test looks for unhealthy levels of porphyrins showing up in the urine. This is a profile indicating damage to the porphyrin pathways specifically because of a mercury body burden. "The test demonstrates the harm being done by mercury because when heme (iron-containing component of hemoglobin that carries oxygen) production is being

[49] The President's Cancer Panel, *Reducing Environmental Cancer Risk* (April 2010), 145.

blocked by mercury, both cellular energy production and oxygen transport in the blood are interfered with."[50]

The test is available at www.metametrix.com.

I believe the MELISA test for sensitivity to metals is important and should be done to determine your individual biocompatibility to any materials placed in your mouth. This test shows sensitization or allergy to metals, including mercury. A reaction to an offending dental material can cause you health problems. You need to do this test in advance so that your dentist will be prepared to use the appropriate materials in your treatment. Visit http://www.melisa.org.

Quicksilver Scientific specializes in mercury speciation. This is an analytical testing process that separates and measures the different forms (species) of mercury that are present in a test sample. Visit www.quicksilverscientific.com.

You may ask why everyone doesn't have problems with any mercury exposure. That is an excellent question.

This has to do with susceptibility to mercury poisoning: "There is great individual variation with regard to susceptibility to mercury. . . . Studies failed to find the characteristic signs and symptom of poisoning as a result of overexposure. This was in spite of the fact that mercury levels in the workers' urine were high (sometimes reaching 500ug/l)."[51]

A factor in the "great individual variation with regard to susceptibility to mercury" has to do with our genetic makeup. It has to do in part with our ability to detoxify mercury from the brain. Apolipoprotein E (APOE) is a gene we inherit from our parents in one of three forms: APOE2, APOE3, or APOE4. APOE2 substantially protects us against Alzheimer's, APOE3 plays a neutral role, and APOE4 dramatically increases the risk of Alzheimer's. About a quarter of Americans have APOE4, while one in twenty has APOE2.

---

50 DAMS, *Dental Truth* (May 2009).

51 Lamm and Pratt, "Sub-Clinical Effects of Exposure," 237–243.

The APOE2 protective effect may have to do with its ability to carry mercury-laden cholesterol out of the brain, while APOE4 has the least protective effect of removing mercury from the brain. Dentists who carry the APOE2 gene would likely be protected more from mercury exposure in general practice.

> "Apolipoprotein-E (APO-E) genotyping has been investigated as an indicator of susceptibility to heavy metal (i.e., lead) neurotoxicity. Moreover, the APO-E epsilon 4 allele is a major risk factor for neuro-degenerative conditions, including Alzheimer's disease (AD)."[52]

Another factor is the protective enzymes. On continued exposure to mercury, these protective enzymes may be used up.[53] Therefore, it is not a good idea to be exposed to mercury from any source, especially mercury-silver fillings, which continually emit mercury. Once these enzymes are depleted or lessened, our bodies would retain more mercury, working havoc on our neurological and immunological systems. This has implications for older people.

Sensitivity has been tested in dental students. This study of dental students showed that by the time they were seniors, the number of dental students who were sensitive to mercury increased. Therefore, it is logical to assume that sensitivity increased with time and exposure.

> "The results of this survey show that there is an increase in the development of hypersensitivity to mercury as students progress through dental school . . . . The fact that the dental students who were the volunteers in this study received only a small fraction of the exposure to mercury that the practicing dentist receives does emphasize the potential of this allergen in actual dental practice."[54]

---

52 Michael E. Godfrey, Damian P. Wojcik, and Cheryl A. Krone, "Apolipoprotein E Genotyping as a Potential Biomarker for Mercury Neurotoxicity," *Journal of Alzheimer's Disease* 5 (2003): 189–195.

53 J. T. A. "Ely, Mercury Induced Alzheimer's Disease: Accelerating Incidence?" *Bull Environ Contam Toxicol* 67 (2001): 800–806.

54 Robert R. White and Robert L. Brandt, "Development of Mercury Hypersensitivity among Dental Students," *JADA* 92 (June 1976): p.

The following factors, therefore, could be the reason some people get sick while others do not:

- Individual susceptibility as determined by genetic makeup.
- Enzyme systems and detoxification mechanisms in the body, which can change.
- Sensitivity, which can develop upon exposure and increase.
- Body burden of mercury: the accumulation of mercury within the brain and the body, which can manifest in any number of neurological and immunological systems. Picture a bathtub filling with water. If the water drains out faster than it is filling, the bathtub will not overflow. If the drain becomes clogged, then the bathtub will overflow and cause problems. It is the same way with mercury in the body. At a certain point, the mercury can become too much for the body to tolerate, depending on the factors listed above. The understanding of mercury toxicity is very complex.

The combination of other heavy metals, such as lead, can cause compounded health problems. Exposure to formaldehyde and mercury can be exponentially more harmful than mercury alone (toxic synergism). Therefore, it might not take too much mercury to cause a severe health problem.

In the book *Explaining "Unexplained Illnesses,"* by Martin L. Pall, PhD, multiple chemical sensitivity (MCS) is discussed.[55] A person becomes so sensitive to many different types of chemicals, including petrochemicals, pesticides, perfumes, etc., that life becomes intolerable. The symptoms vary from agonizing irritability to headaches, insomnia, asthma, and various other disorders. Sometimes it is hard to determine the toxic material that caused the problem. There is no doubt in my mind that mercury is one of the triggers of this problem. As I have a documented history of chronic mercury toxicity, it is the cause of my MCS.

1206.

[55] Martin L. Pall, PhD, "Explaining "Unexplained Illnesses"", (2009), 116-134.

The effect of mercury can be very subtle. In the book, *The Edge Effect*, by Eric R. Braverman, MD, brain neurotransmitters are discussed. Chemicals in our environment can make us "edgy or nervous."[56] Lead is mentioned as a heavy metal that can disturb brain function. Since mercury is much more neurotoxic than lead, insidious neuropsychological problems can result. This leads to the possibility that your fillings can make you more irritable and affect the way you feel. Can you imagine what a boon this is to the pharmaceutical industry with all the ads on treatments for depression, insomnia, and other neurological disorders?

---

[56] Eric R. Braverman, The Edge Effect (Sterling, 2004), 135.

Chapter 23

Replacing Mercury-Silver Fillings

It is important to be aware of the problem of mercury-silver fillings. We should take precautions and limit our exposure to mercury. We need to be aware of the various sources of mercury exposure, including fish and especially mercury-silver fillings.

It is especially important for women of childbearing age not to have any exposure to mercury as it can be passed on to the developing baby in utero and breastfeeding. Removal of mercury-silver fillings causes high mercury exposure and must be done way in advance of having a family. This should be done under the supervision of a knowledgeable physician and dentist. Be sure that any required vaccinations are performed without thimerosal, a mercury preservative in vaccines. Although thimerosal has been removed from childhood vaccines, it is still present in adult flu shots.

My friend Pat asked me, "How do you find a dentist who can properly replace mercury-silver fillings?"

First, I would ask the dentist if he places mercury-silver fillings. If he says, "Yes," run! Today, the modern dentist uses cosmetic restorative materials such as composite and porcelain. More than 50 percent of dentists are no longer using mercury-silver fillings. A dentist who is no longer using these archaic pre–civil war fillings has more experience with the state-of-the-art composites and porcelain restorations. These restorations require a more exacting technique as compared to mercury-silver fillings. In addition, a dentist using the newer cosmetic materials is more likely to be aware of the potential toxicity of mercury-silver fillings.

While you still have mercury-silver fillings, it is important not to place any metallic materials, such as gold. Gold crowns and inlays can increase the galvanic effect in the mouth, drawing out more mercury. The mouth is like a battery where electric currents can be measured. The more current there is from a mercury-silver filling, the more mercury ions are coming out.

Next, especially if you believe you have some unexplained medical problems, you would want to find a dentist who is trained in proper removal and replacement of amalgams. You would want to avoid high exposure to mercury when these fillings are ground out. To give you an idea of the possible medical complaints associated with mercury exposure, complete the medical questionnaire form at the end of this book. The more symptoms in multiple categories you have in this questionnaire, the more you should be suspicious of a systemic poison.

Caution: It is generally a good idea to remove and replace amalgam (mercury) fillings, but only if it is done by a well-trained and well-equipped dentist who can do it safely, with elaborate protections.

There are no guarantees that you will get better if you have a mercury-related problem. However, many people have had improved health.

The following table might give you an idea of the probabilities of relief. 1569 patients participated in this study.[57]

[57] Bioprobe Newsletter, March, 1993.

Symptom Reported	Percentage of patients claiming substantial relief
Allergy	89%
Anxiety	93
Bad temper	89
Bloating	88
Blood pressure problems	54
Chest pains	87
Depression	91
Dizziness	88
Fatigue	86
Gastrointestinal problems	83
Gum problems	94
Headaches	87
Migraine	87
Insomnia	78
Irregular heartbeat	87
Irritibility	90
Lack of concentration	80
Lack of energy	97
Memory loss	73
Metallic taste	95
Multiple sclerosis	76
Muscle tremor	83
Nervousness	83
Numbness	82
Skin disturbances	81
Sore throat	86
Tachycardia	70
Thyroid problems	79
Oral ulcers	86

Urinary tract problems	76
Vision problems	63

It is advisable to consult with your dentist regarding any risks, such as replacement of a deep filling. In a tooth with weak walls, consideration should be made whether to place a porcelain onlay on the tooth. This will help prevent a wall from shearing and causing a crack in the tooth. I can tell you I lost a few teeth from fracturing because they did not have the protection of an onlay.

Please obtain more information from the sources below for assistance:

Dentists and patients can consult with the International Academy of Oral Medicine and Toxicology for advice. The academy has courses and information for dentists and assists dental patients.

Call the International Academy of Oral Medicine and Toxicology at 863-420-6373, or visit their website at http://www.iaomt.org/ for more information. Here you will find information on safe amalgam removal. Download the document "Safe Removal of Amalgam Fillings." The Academy can direct patients to members who are properly trained in amalgam removal and replacement.

Also, call DAMS (Dental Amalgam Mercury Solutions) at 651-644-4572 for assistance, or visit http://www.flcv.com/dams.html.

Dr. Hal Huggins Internet site has information on mercury and detoxification protocol: www.DrHuggins.com Dr. Huggins includes in his protocol sequential removal of the mercury fillings. This requires that the quadrant containing the highest negative current filling be removed first. Then the quadrant with the next highest electrical charge is next. I personally feel that sequential amalgam removal should be done although there are practitioners who do not feel it is necessary. Nutritional supplementation in addition to chelation should be considered as there may be an imbalance of minerals, etc. due to mercury.

Candida albicans, a yeast form, is often a problem due to mercury exposure. Mercury acts like an antibiotic in destroying beneficial symbiotic bacteria in the intestines. With the destruction of the good bacteria such as lactobacillus, Candida tends to overgrow in the intestine and become pathological. Its cells become elongated (mycelial form) allowing it to penetrate into living tissue and cause many problems. The use of probiotics to replenish the good bacteria in the intestines is helpful. Even though mercury may be eliminated as a cause, there may be lingering health problems due to Candida albicans.

Some techniques for safe removal of amalgam fillings:

- The patient can breathe through the nose-piece of a tank of medical air, avoiding inhaling the amalgam dust and mercury vapor.
- High-volume air vacuum system or an ionizing system can be used to clean the mercury vapor out of the air in the office.
- Dentist and assistant can use a respirator to limit their own mercury exposure while cutting out an old amalgam.
- High-speed suction should be used by an assistant at all times during removal of fillings.
- Use a nitrile rubber dam or, alternatively, the "Clean-Up" suction tip. Contact IAOMT at 863-420-6373 or http://www.iaomt.org/ or DAMS at 651-644-4572.
- With constant water spray, cut amalgam out in sections rather than completely grinding the amalgam. This will reduce the amount of amalgam dust. The dust can imbed itself deeply in the lungs where mercury can be released.

The elaborate precautions in "Safe Removal of Amalgam Fillings" will serve to protect both the dental personnel and the dental patient.

If there is a possible mercury problem, a health professional knowledgeable on the subject can guide you with supplementation to help your body detoxify.

DMSA and DMPS are recognized to chelate mercury. These should be used under the care of your health practitioner. These compounds are sulfur bearing and have the ability to bind and eliminate mercury from the body. Sulfur has a strong affinity for mercury.

There are nutritional supplements that can help the body eliminate mercury. Dr. Robert Jay Rowen recommends a cocktail of nutrients. It includes selenium (200 mcg daily), N-acetyl-cysteine (500 mg, 3 times daily), alpha lipoic acid (300 mg daily), and vitamin C (1,000 mg, 2 to 3 times daily). In addition, he has used dl-methionine (100 mg daily), although he says that the first four nutrients are the mainstay. He reports that this inexpensive combination has reduced overall body burden based on DMPS challenge in virtually everyone he has treated, often in as little as three months but virtually always in nine months, as long as amalgams are gone. If not, this combination can protect against damage from continuing mercury release. This combination of nutrients helps raise glutathione levels, which is the body's natural detoxifier.[58]

Another natural ingredient that helps detoxify mercury from the body is chlorella. Chlorella is a blue-green alga.[59]

OSR (Oxidative stress relief) is a fat-soluble antioxidant and helps increase glutathione. Regarding OSR, Christopher Shade, in the *Dental Truth* newsletter, January 2010, page 13, stated that his testing showed "OSR's structure makes a great complexing agent for mercury, especially for inorganic mercury."

OSR is a very safe and strong chelator of mercury, lead, cadmium, and arsenic. In experiments on rats injected with multiple lethal doses of mercury, the injection of OSR twenty minutes later caused complete recovery from mercury toxicity. OSR is also an extremely potent antioxidant. So just as glutathione is used by the body to chelate and remove mercury and, as a major antioxidant, to protect against hydroxyl radical formation, OSR behaves in the same manner, only much more effective. As of this date, the FDA has taken this product off

---

[58] Robert J. Rowen, *Second Opinion Newsletter*, September 2010, www.secondopinionnewsletter.com.

[59] Ibid.

the market. Although CTI Science did not make any medical claims on their product, there were quite a few people on the Internet who stated that they had been getting relief from medical problems. The FDA, thereupon, stated that OSR is a drug and requires proper scientific investigation before being released back on the market. I understand that OSR may become available again under another name in 2013. www.ctiscience.com

I had been taking OSR for about four months, and I feel it has helped me quite a bit. I had fewer attacks of internal tremors and agitation. I call it amazing because in the many years that I have been trying to obtain relief from my agony, there has been nothing else as effective! Since OSR is no longer available, my tremors have come back intermittently.

If you believe you have a health related mercury problem, you should coordinate your treatment with your dentist and knowledgeable health care practitioner. Recommendations can be made by the International Academy of Oral Medicine and Toxicology (863-420-6373).

Chapter 24

Rip van Winkle

It was like waking up from a bad dream. What I thought would be several months to recover, or even a year, turned out to be more than twenty years since 1984, when I had to give up my dental practice. The torturous, agonizing morbid irritability-agitation with the internal tremors was letting up. The years had passed by, but I had hung on. But now, I was better!

I had been in an altered state of consciousness, living through a nightmare. It had been a surreal existence, as if I was a part of a weird movie. What I had gone through was so unreal: the claustrophobia, the fear of heights, the inability to stand loud noises or excitement in a movie, the fear of flying, and more. I had never had these feelings prior to my mercury illness. I had been so caught up in the deluge of my illness that I could not really appreciate all that was around me. I had felt that through the chatter of my disrupted brain "circuitry," God could not hear me. Perhaps now, my prayers to God could be heard. The intense vibrations were letting up, and there were finally times when they were not noticeable. One time, I cried in gratefulness for the temporary relief.

As my preoccupation of being caught up in this terrible nightmare and illness began to fade, I was left with the issue of what was I going to do without the profession I was so good at. I was concerned about income since money was very tight without my dental practice.

The days seemed to disappear in a blur. The days turned into months, and then into years. My marriage was suffering as my wife had lost her respect for me. She used to tell me that it was not my fault, but she wanted me to be productive again. I really did not know where to turn. I was about forty-six years old when I gave up my dental practice. Then I was in my sixties. Although feeling better, I still had health deficits and was still disabled. We both hung on to our marriage for two reasons: the first was keeping our family together for our sons, and the other was financial. I remember Dr. Hal Huggins saying that he knew very few marriages had survived mercury toxicity in a spouse. I thought ours would be the exception.

Nicole* was a nutritionist, a French lady with a kind heart. She had heard about my problem and contacted me. She had sent me some type of device to try to help. She did this without expecting any reimbursement. She just wanted to help. She and her husband, Bob*, later moved to Florida, where I met her. She introduced me to Joe*, who had problems similar to mine. Through the years, Joe and I have talked about our conditions.

We tried to examine Joe's exposure to mercury. As a marine diver, he was exposed to more mercury from his silver fillings than the average person because of his work doing electric welding underwater. The following documentation explains his increased exposure to mercury:

- Electrical activity is generated during the process of electric welding or cutting under water. This activity was not considered at a high-enough magnitude to cause a problem. However, "a metallic taste and a subjective change in the diver's dental amalgam were provoked."
- "An increased surface deterioration of dental amalgam was detected in those divers who had performed electrical welding/ cutting during the previous two years."

- "The flux density of the intraoral magnetic field created by a current of 650 ADC was calculated and measured to be 1.15 mT, which is approximately 25 times stronger than that of the earth. When exposing divers in-vivo to a field generated by a 200 ADC current, no symptoms other than magnetophosphenes were reported, such as metallic taste. The divers' helmets offered almost no shielding effect towards the magnetic field. In-vitro exposure of dental amalgams to a magnetic field (1.15 mT; 50 Hz) increased the mobility of copper and especially mercury in the superficial layers of the amalgam after 24 h exposure, and gave rise to slight morphological changes within the amalgam."[60]

Just the very fact that the fillings were breaking down indicates the loss of mercury from the surface. The article states increased mobilization of mercury. If the average minimum vaporization of a mercury-silver filling is 10 mcg/day, then the increased breakdown of these fillings would create a higher vaporization level. In this document, however, they did not find any "increased levels of mercury or copper in the saliva, blood, or urine." There must be a reason for this. Perhaps the transfer of mercury ions to tissue may be higher under a magnetic field, making it too transient to be detected in bodily fluids. The mercury has to go somewhere!

Joe was involved in the importing and marketing business. In his warehouse, he was exposed to formaldehyde from imported products. In one of my lectures on mercury, Dr. Max Daunderer, a clinical toxicologist, stated that exposure to formaldehyde greatly multiplies the effect of mercury toxicity in the body (synergistic toxicity). This could help explain the sudden and mysterious health deterioration that ensued. Joe became so chemically sensitive that he could not live in a normal environment. He found a place in Florida with minimal pollution. I must respect Joe for his unbelievable discipline to survive. He told me that when you're sick enough, you have no choice. We both have been searching for answers so that we could be normal again.

---

[60] T. Ortendahl, "Oral Changes in Divers Working with Electrical Welding/Cutting Underwater," *Swed Dent J Suppl* 43 (1987): 1–53.

I have included the above story for physicians and divers who have a history of electric welding and/or cutting underwater and unusual medical problems. Perhaps I can help someone with this information.

Multiple Chemical Sensitivity (MCS)

MCS can develop for many reasons. It is usually caused by some type of a severe toxic condition. In my case, it was clearly due to my mercury illness. This syndrome can be caused by the mercury derived from mercury-silver fillings. When the accumulation of mercury in the body exceeds a certain tolerance level, a person may become chemically sensitive to many different agents.

I had to be careful what I ate. If I had a wheat cereal in the morning, I would go through a few hours of agitation. It was difficult to think during these times. I became extremely sensitive to any fumes. Petrochemicals, insecticides, and perfumes give me a headache and sets off these internal vibrations with agitation.

Just as I was writing the above paragraph, I received a phone call from a representative of Allergy Research. Dr. Stephen Levine's story of how he overcame multiple chemical sensitivity is really amazing. The last time I spoke to him was about twenty years ago; I told him my story and asked him for advice. Receiving a call from Dr. Levine's representative, who came to see me within a few minutes, was unbelievable timing.

One time, in front of my Siesta Key house, there were hundreds of ants. I took out the Raid aerosol can and sprayed the ants. I held my breath so as not to inhale any of the fumes. I walked away and started breathing normally. I walked back to the area to see if I had gotten all the ants. I took two normal breaths, sensed the fumes, and walked away. I became terribly sick again. During that time, I wondered if I would ever get better. In about a month, the agitation lessened. I was so grateful that it was over.

I had another major setback with a pesticide application in my house. A pest control man, Ray*, knew my history of mercury poisoning and chemical sensitivity. He explained to me that he would only use diatomaceous earth in my home, which was safe for me. I trusted Ray and let no other pest control company in my house, knowing the danger that I could be exposed to. Then I had a terrible reaction. I asked him to treat the bathroom for bugs. Without my authorization, his associate applied pesticide to my whole house. I later found out that it was not diatomaceous earth but another product. My house became uninhabitable for me. I felt as though I was dying. Have you ever seen a spider shrivel up after being sprayed with Raid?

I reported my reaction to the pesticide application to the Florida Department of Entomology and Pest Control. Their investigation proved to be worse than what I thought. It was not just a case of chemical sensitivity but actual poisoning. This pesticide company inadvertently used a chemical inside my house, *Termidor SC*, against label directions. I had a relapse for over six months.

Perhaps people who are chemically sensitive are like canaries in a coal mine who could warn of possible danger. Pesticides, heavy metals, and petrochemicals are potentially dangerous. Just because we don't react to them doesn't mean that they cannot wreak havoc on our health. As people are living longer, there is much degenerative illness. Can we reduce illness by reducing our exposure to these toxic chemicals? I think we can, and there are many others in preventive medicine who also think that way.

I especially think of Dr. Garry Gordon (http://www.gordonresearch.com). Dr. Gordon is a world-recognized authority on chelation therapy and environmental medicine. His focus is treating the cause, not masking the symptoms with a drug. He leads a large forum of health professionals. His company, Longevity Plus, which can be contacted at 800-580-7587, provides chelating agents that help remove mercury from the body. He states that "everyone today has potentially dangerous levels of toxins including lead and mercury which most experts agree can interfere with enzyme functions that are vital for repair and detoxification of every cell in the body."

Chapter 25

Ending Notes

Like in the movie *The NeverEnding Story*, this book is not just about me; it is ultimately about you, the dentist, and the patient. Mercury is the most neurotoxic non-radioactive element known to man. It is so insidious that it is virtually impossible to diagnose medically related problems using classical methods.

We are all in some way being exposed to mercury. It may be from mercury-silver fillings, vaccinations, and fish. The air and environment may become contaminated by coal-burning facilities, alkali and metal processing, mining of gold and mercury, and medical and other wastes. Natural sources of atmospheric mercury include volcanoes, geologic deposits of mercury, and volatilization from the ocean. Once in the atmosphere, mercury can remain in the air for many years and cause wide distribution over the land.[61]

The increased use of fluorescent lights containing mercury as an energy conservation measure leads to increased mercury exposure. Compact fluorescent lights (CFLs) have become very popular lately because they help save electricity. Not everyone disposes of used fluorescent lights

---

61 http://www.usgs.gov/themes/factsheet/146-00/

properly, and this adds to mercury in our environment. These used lights should be taken to a recycling facility so that the environment is not contaminated. Fluorescent lights present a serious hazard when they break in your house since mercury is released.

Our country and many other countries obtain a great deal of energy from coal-burning facilities. The contaminated air from coal burning makes its way around the globe. China burns a huge amount of coal for its energy needs. Mercury from China can make its way eastward to the West Coast of the United States. Countries are no longer isolated as what one country does can affect other countries. We are all connected.

It has been documented that the primary body burden in the human population is mercury derived from mercury-silver fillings. Fortunately, more than 50 percent of dentists are not using these fillings anymore. But hundreds of millions of people have already had this deadly material implanted in their teeth.

Sweden has banned the use of mercury in dentistry. As of this date, in 2011, the Food and Drug Administration still allows the use of this toxic material.

It seems that the EPA and the FDA are concerned about women "who may become pregnant, pregnant women, nursing mothers, and young children" being exposed to mercury from fish. These are two of their recommendations:

1. Do not eat shark, swordfish, king mackerel, or tilefish because they contain high levels of mercury.
2. Eat up to twelve ounces (two average meals) a week of a variety of fish and shellfish that are lower in mercury.

Five of the most commonly eaten fish that are low in mercury are shrimp, canned light tuna, salmon, pollock, and catfish. Another commonly eaten fish, albacore ("white") tuna, has more mercury than canned light tuna. So when choosing your two meals of fish and shellfish, you may eat up to six ounces (one average meal) of albacore tuna per week. Visit http://www.epa.gov/fishadvisories/advice/.

Then what about the mercury from mercury-silver fillings?

The following is an article that I wrote for the *Sarasota Herald-Tribune in 2009*:

> "In 1978 Congress ordered the FDA to require that all medical and dental devices be classified (to reflect their safety and efficacy) based on sound scientific evidence. In a shocking recent announcement, certain FDA officials rejected dozens of peer-reviewed research studies documenting significant human health risks posed by mercury derived from dental fillings.
>
> The FDA has now classified a filling containing mercury—which has been declared by the Environmental Protection Agency a toxic waste disposal hazard! —as a class II dental device, meaning that the FDA is claiming that it carries only a moderate risk. This is despite the FDA's own current advisories that pregnant women should limit their dietary intake of certain fish due to their mercury content—even though studies have shown that mercury dental fillings contribute two to three times as much mercury to the human body as air, dietary and environmental sources combined.
>
> Even as more and more devastating neurological and other disorders continue to be linked to mercury, the FDA—the federal agency entrusted by Congress and the American public to advise and protect us from harmful products—assures us that this particular source of mercury, the most potent neuro-toxic element on earth, is safe even for pregnant women and children."

The following is a summary of a document from Charles G. Brown, national counsel for Consumers for Dental Choice:

"President Obama came into office promising to improve United States health care." As a candidate, he promised to reduce mercury's health risks. When Democrats returned to power, Hamburg ascended to FDA commissioner. Hamburg was formally employed by the Henry Schein Dental Company, the largest distributor of mercury in dentistry.

Hamburg was paid lavishly by the dental products distributor Henry Schein Inc. She continued to own Schein stock options even after becoming commissioner. While still having a financial interest in the Schein Dental Company, she made a ruling on dental amalgam. The rule favored her benefactor Henry Schein Inc. "The rule allows amalgam to be sold without disclosing to consumers that it contains mercury." It is amazing that the FDA bans mercury in all veterinary products yet allows the use of mercury in fillings even in little children, who are most vulnerable. "The new FDA, under Margaret Hamburg and her Sancho Panza, Joshua Sharfstein, have decided that children don't merit the protection FDA gives horses and dogs."[62]

I believe Commissioner Hamburg's decision on mercury-silver fillings is a disappointment to President Obama, who wants to improve the health care system for the citizens of the United States.

Money and power seem to be in control. One of my goals in this book is to make the public aware of a very serious insidious problem. For the public, knowledge is power, and together we can make a difference. We can fight corruption and biased interests that go against the health and welfare of the public. We can make our elected officials know of our concerns and demand that we get the proper protection.

If we are to have a viable health care system, we need to stop poisoning our people. This may be politically inconvenient for the American Dental Association and may reduce profits for the dental mercury manufactures. However, many people have had their health impaired by this insidious poison. Many more people will be health impaired if the use of mercury-silver dental fillings continues.

Evidently, the risk of mercury is known. On January 24, 2012, President Obama gave the State of the Union address: "We will not back down from protecting our kids from mercury pollution, or making sure that our food is safe and our water is clean."

---

[62] Charles G. Brown, Consumers for Dental Choice, August 6, 2009.

Chapter 26

Reflections

You may have heard of the Mad Hatter. Lewis Carroll popularized this character in his book *Alice's Adventures in Wonderland*. Mercury was used to process felt hats during the time his book was written. The phrase "mad as a hatter" has been used to associate the effects of mercury on behavior, mood swings, and other toxic effects.

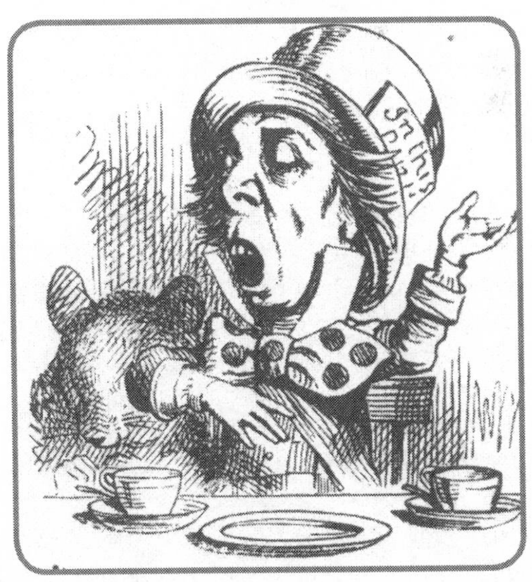

Many people have heard about mercury in silver fillings. People know about the issue but are not really sure. Many dentists who are wary about mercury are not even fully aware of the science on the toxicity of these fillings. Here, I have presented my life story and the science to go along with it.

The first major exposé of the amalgam controversy was aired on TV on December 16, 1990, on CBS with Morley Safer. The show *60 Minutes* did an exposé on mercury-silver fillings. Thirty million people watched this program. The American Dental Association immediately went into damage control, sending information to its membership. Usually, *60 Minutes* airs their programs twice. This program on mercury was not aired for a second time.

Evidently, there is a lot of money involved, and there are interests that do not want this story told. In fact, I had visited Dr. Joel Berger, who is now an attorney, after he had lost his New York state dental license for being vocal regarding the amalgam issue. He said to me that my book should be named *The Story That Must Be Told!*

Dr. Boyd Haley, a leading scientist on mercury toxicology, who very clearly sees the issue from the perspective of science, has met much opposition in trying to stop the use of mercury in dentistry. Other countries have taken steps to eliminate mercury from medicine and dentistry. The United States is severely lacking in this regard.

In a press release from the government offices of Sweden dated January 15, 2009, the Ministry of the Environment, the following was stated: "Government bans all use of mercury in Sweden, The Government today decided to introduce a blanket ban on mercury. The ban means that the use of dental amalgam in fillings will cease and that it will no longer be permitted to place products containing mercury on the Swedish market." Other countries are taking steps to protect the public. The United States should do so too!

I believe that we dentists, as a professional group, are held in the highest esteem by the public. I know my colleagues want to do the right thing for their patients. In order to do so, they need to learn the facts and the science. It is not enough for them to hear the side that says that it would take three hundred fillings for any problem to arise. At a minimum of 10 mcg/daily of mercury from a filling, it does not take too many fillings for a person to be at risk. Three hundred fillings would be an unbelievably large amount.

The first year of dental school should have courses in toxicology and immunology related to the dental procedures that we perform. We need to be aware that the materials used in dentistry can affect our health. These dental materials need to be biocompatible with our body so that it does not tax our immune system.

The health condition of the mouth can affect the rest of the body. Infections can spread from the mouth to other tissues and organs. Bacteria from the mouth can be a source of bacteria to other parts of the body. A healthy mouth is important for a healthy body.

The Internet is replete with information on mercury in silver fillings. With the information explosion on the Internet, knowledge in a free society cannot be held back. Although powerful interests can control the media, still, the public has free access to information. All you have to do is type in the words *silver fillings*, *mercury fillings*, etc., into an Internet search engine, and you will get both sides of the story. After reading my book, you can judge the position of the mercury advocates. You can see what makes most sense to you. Do a Google search on Dr. David Kennedy and mercury. He has some great Internet videos. He has been very helpful to me through the years. He has been a valuable source of information for me.

Even as dental amalgam, this "sin against humanity", disappears into oblivion, this is not the end of the story about mercury; this is just the the beginning.

> "The climate that is changing the most is an advancing bio-accumulating mass of mercury pollution, which is literally contaminating everything on the planet. It's mercury that is the real danger coming out of the smokestacks of the industrialized world not CO2 but the people up on top do not want the public focused on one of the greatest threats to human well being that exists."
>
> Dr. Mark Sircus

Mercury pollution in our environment contaminates every living organism on earth. Allopathic medicine seems oblivious to a major cause of many degenerative illnesses which can be related to pollution of many different toxins acting synergistically. Metabolic medicine will be the future wave of modern rational treatment. They will look at the cause of the problem rather than just trying to mask the symptoms with petroleum based pharmaceuticals.

> "Because mercury is increasingly becoming elevated in all forms of life, we can assume that more people will have some defects in pancreatic function. Pancreatic support is increasingly necessary for optimal health."
>
> Dr. Garry Gordon

The beta cells of the pancreas produce insulin. When the function of the pancreas and glucose metabolism is compromised, diabetes can be the result. According to an article in WebMD News Archive, a diabetes epidemic will hit half of the U.S. by 2020. We need to be addressing the cause for such illnesses, not just put more people on insulin. Reducing exposure to toxic materials and assisting the body to eliminate toxins should be an important consideration.

A plea for preventive medicine: I am reminded of a poem about an ambulance and a fence on top of a cliff. People were falling off the cliff, and the town had to decide what to do. Should they go through the expense of constructing a fence, or should they just keep going on taking the injured people who fell off the cliff to the hospital by ambulance. If they left things the way they were, the hospital would continue to make a lot of money, and the patients would pay a high price for this medical care. If a fence were placed, people would be spared their suffering and medical costs.

What are we going to do as a people? Let's stop using this archaic vile poisonous material in dentistry! Let's make a change together!

The question that I have for myself is, can I make a difference? Can I help people who have an iatrogenic (medically caused) illness? Can I help prevent more people from being hurt? Can my years of suffering be for a reason? I pray for a change in our health care system that works by *prevention, by not poisoning the public.* This in itself will make medical care more affordable.

About fifty years ago, cigarette manufacturers were advertising in the *Journal of the American Medical Association* and in leading American magazines. The headlines read, "More Doctors Smoke Camels than Any Other Cigarette!" Fifty years from now, will the use of mercury in dentistry, the most toxic non-radioactive element known to man, be remembered the same way?

I am a dreamer. I see a world free of pollution. I see a world with abundant energy through solar, wind, and unlimited hydrogen fusion power. I see a world where nation shall not lift sword against nation, and there shall be war no more. We do not have a choice, and this is the way it must be for us to survive.

I have been a science fiction fan, especially of Isaac Asimov. There were lines in the beginning of one of his books that I read over forty years ago that are still in my mind today. I have hung onto this hope through all this time from when I was a young man:

"Grow old along with me,

The best is yet to be!"

I hope the journey that I have taken you on will make a difference!

Appendix

Medical Questionnaire

Please check all past or present symptoms that apply to you.

1. Heart Problems

___ heart/chest pains
___ angina
___ tachycardia
___ heart murmur
___ low blood pressure
___ abnormal EKG
___ endocarditis
___ partial heart block
___ high blood pressure
___ heart attack

2. Skin Problems

___ unexplained rashes
___ excessive itching
___ red flushes of color
___ rough skin
___ acne (pimples)

3. Nervous Disorders

___ Bell's palsy
___ multiple sclerosis
___ shingles
___ epilepsy/convulsions
___ Dr. told you "it's your nerves"
___ the shakes of hands, feet, head, etc.
___ twitching of face or other muscles

4. Digestion

___ diverticulitis
___ ulcers
___ Crohn's disease
___ Graves' disease
___ indigestion
___ diarrhea
___ bloated feeling after eating
___ heartburn
___ poor appetite
___ diarrhea

5. Blood Disease

___ mononucleosis
___ false positive for venereal disease

6. Cancer

___ leukemia
___ Hodgkin's disease
___ any other name

7. Endocrine Problems

___ diabetes
___ ovaries
___ hysterectomy – complete
___ tipped uterus
___ overweight
___ thyroid overactive
___ testes
___ pancreas
___ cervical erosion
___ underweight
___ prostate
___ menstruation – painful, too often, or too seldom/ stopping without reason

8. Emotional

___ sudden anger
___ depression
___ wish you were dead
___ irritability
___ suicidal tendencies
___ been divorced

9. Annoying Symptoms

___ frequent headaches
___ noises in your ears
___ ringing in your ears
___ hissing in your ears
___ chronic eye inflammation
___ chronic fatigue
___ do you tire easily?
___ swollen lymph nodes
___ do you sweat excessively?
___ hearing problems
___ cold hands and feet
___ motion sickness
___ slow healing
___ leg cramps
___ dizziness
___ get up at night to urinate
___ urinate frequently during the day
___ have insomnia
___ tired when awaken in the morning
___ have trouble making decisions

10. Allergies

___ metal
___ fabrics
___ soaps and detergents
___ food
___ other

11. Diseases

___ rheumatoid
___ bursitis
___ tennis elbow
___ painful joints
___ Friedreich's ataxia
___ asthma
___ surgery (for what?)
___ osteomyelitis
___ psoriasis
___ sickle-cell anemia
___ chronic anemia
___ kidney stones

12. Miscellaneous

___ infections take a long time to heal

___ do you work around mercury, what capacity?

___ what medications are you taking?

13. Dental History

___ had silver amalgams
___ have silver amalgams
___ had gold fillings
___ have gold fillings now
___ removable metal bridge
___ gold bridge
___ porcelain caps (crowns)
___ non-precious crowns
___ root canal
___ root canal now
___ metallic taste in mouth
___ burning sensation in mouth
___ increased flow of saliva

We are grateful to Dr. Hal Huggins for the above questionnaire. The checklist may assist in evaluating mercury toxicity.

Made in the USA
San Bernardino, CA
24 October 2017